MW00763610

The Brain   *NEW SERIES

Edited By: Helen Dwyer
Curriculum Connections: Psychology
Series of 6
Black Rabbit Books/Brown Bear Books Imprint
978-1-936333-16-5
$39.95 (List) each
$27.95 (School/Library) each
112 pages
Reading Level: Grades 10 and up
Color Photographs and Illustrations, Labeled Diagrams, Charts,
Curriculum Context sidebars, Glossary within text
Release date: March, 2011

This comprehensive series for high school students examines every
aspect of the science of psychology. Fundamental concepts are
explored in detail and their importance and relevance is explained as
well. Extensive use of full-color, detailed illustrations and labeled
diagrams throughout the volumes complement the thorough text.

Why did we publish this series?

This series makes use of "curriculum context" sidebars, an innovative
feature that tells students why the information they are reading is
important, how it links to other curriculum topics, and thus helps them
prepare for tests. This unique feature helps provide students with
immediate context and is a valuable aid in comprehension and
retention of subject matter. Teachers will find this feature a valuable
resource as well.

Curriculum Connections: Psychology

Titles in this series:
Abnormal Psychology
The Brain
Cognitive Development
The History of Psychology
Intellectual Development
The Individual and Society

Contact Information:
Ann Schwab
Black Rabbit Books
P.O. Box 3263
Mankato, MN 56002
507.388.1633
aschwab@blackrabbitbooks.com

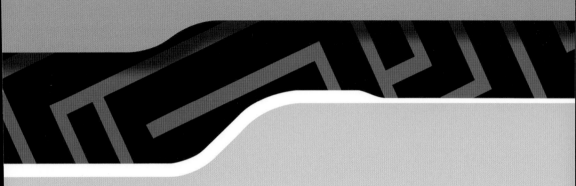

Psychology

The Brain

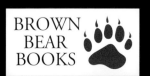

BROWN
BEAR
BOOKS

Published by Brown Bear Books Limited

4877 N. Circulo Bujia
Tucson
AZ 85718
USA

First Floor
9–17 St. Albans Place
London N1 0NX
UK

www.brownreference.com

ISBN: 978-1-936333-16-5

Editorial Director: Lindsey Lowe
Managing Editor: Tim Cooke
Project Director: Laura Durman
Editor: Helen Dwyer
Designer: Barry Dwyer
Picture Researcher: Barry Dwyer

Library of Congress Cataloging-in-Publication Data available upon request

Picture Credits

Cover Image
Shutterstock: idesign

Shutterstock: pp. 6 (Scott Rothstein), 36 (Triff), 38 (Ekaterina Starshaya), 45 (Lisa F. Young), 56 (mphot), 65 (nialat), 71 (zhu difeng), 75 (B. Speckart), 81 (Myron Pronyshyn), 82 (gallimaufry), 84 (Laurin Rinder), 88 (Pauline Breijer), 93 (Dallas Events Inc), 94 (Konstantin Sutyagin), 97 (Karin Hildebrand Lau), 98 (Serhiy Kobyakov), 102 (astroskeptic), 104 (Galyna Andrushko); Wikimedia Commons: pp. 13 (Ökologix), 29, 32, 40 (Erik Charlton), 43 (Giovanni Dall'Orto)

Artwork © The Brown Reference Group Ltd

The Brown Reference Group Ltd has made every effort to trace copyright holders of the pictures used in this book. Anyone having claims to ownership not identified above is invited to contact The Brown Reference Group Ltd.

Printed in the United States of America

Contents

Introduction

Psychology forms part of the Curriculum Connections series. Each of the six volumes of the set covers a particular aspect of psychology: History of Psychology; The Brain; Cognitive Development; Intellectual Development; The Individual and Society; and Abnormal Psychology.

About this set

Each volume in *Psychology* features illustrated chapters, providing in-depth information about each subject. The chapters are all listed in the contents pages of each book. Each volume can be studied to provide a comprehensive understanding of the different aspects of psychology. However, each chapter may also be studied independently.

Within each chapter there are two key aids to learning that are to be found in color sidebars located in the margins of each page:

Curriculum Context sidebars indicate to the reader that a subject has a particular relevance to certain key state and national psychology guidelines and curricula. They highlight essential information or suggest useful ways for students to consider a subject or to include it in their studies.

Glossary sidebars define key words within the text.

At the end of the book, a summary **Glossary** lists the key terms defined in the volume. There is also a list of further print and Web-based resources and a full volume index.

Fully captioned illustrations play an important role throughout the set, including photographs and explanatory diagrams.

About this book

The Brain analyzes the many theories that have been proposed regarding the brain, and looks in detail at how this vital organ works.

The first chapter, History of the Brain, examines how our understanding of the brain and mind has developed over many centuries. Scientists began examining the brain in detail in Europe from the 15th century. Today, we have an in-depth understanding of the brain and its workings, along with its historical evolution.

In Biology of the Brain, the anatomy of this complex organ is examined. The chapter provides an in-depth description of the brain and its regions, with details of the role that each part plays in controlling conscious and unconscious thoughts and actions.

The volume goes on to analyze the concept of the mind as an intagible and invisible entity and the relationship between the mind and the brain. It also investigates how our perceptual systems—eyes, ears, nose, tongue, and other sensors—work to interpret the sensations we experience and how the brain translates information that the sensors produce.

Since ancient times people have attempted to explain what emotions are, how they are caused, and which parts of the brain coordinate them. Emotion and Motivation examines the role that emotions play in both mental health and our everyday lives.

The final chapter looks closely at the concept of consciousness. Many theories have been offered to explain it, from the purely philosophical to those based on neuropsychology and even artificial intelligence. While there has been much progress in recent years, no real consensus has been reached about the nature of consciousness.

History of the Brain

Historical records suggest that ancient civilizations did not recognize the importance of the brain. It was not until the European Renaissance that the brain was examined in detail, and it was only in the latter part of the 20th century that scientists formalized their understanding of how the brain works.

More than 100 years ago archaeologists and paleontologists excavated human skulls dating back to the Stone Age. The skulls showed clear indications of primitive surgery—holes drilled in the upper forehead into the frontal lobes of the brain. No one can be sure why these operations, known as trephinations, were done. Some scientists believe that trephinations were performed on men who had sustained serious head injuries in battle. Yet another theory suggests that the operation was an attempt to remove harmful spirits from the body: the holes were bored to let the evil spirits out. Whatever the reason for these operations, it is clear that many patients survived. More than half of the skulls show signs of healing.

Egyptian understanding
The first known use of the term *neuro* appears in an Egyptian document from about 1700 B.C. It was possibly written by the Egyptian physician Imhotep, who had been studying texts dating from 3000 B.C. In it are accounts of 48 surgical cases, some of which

Ancient Egyptians believed that mummification would keep the person's life force alive. A death mask was sometimes made of the face, and some internal organs were preserved, but the brain was discarded as it was believed to be of little significance.

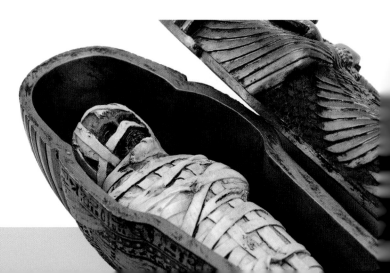

include discussion of the structure of the brain as well as a wider description of the central nervous system. The surgeon clearly describes the linings, or meninges, that protect the brain and cerebrospinal fluid, which protects the delicate brain tissues and spinal cord.

Greek and Roman advances

The Greek physician Hippocrates (c.460–c.377 B.C.) described the relationship between the brain and epilepsy. This was the first true discussion on the nature and functions of the brain.

Epilepsy
A disorder marked by convulsions or periods of loss of consciousness.

The Greek physician and philosopher Galen (A.D. 129–c.199) produced a vast amount of literature on medicine and the medical practices of the time. Observation was the key to Galen's method, and his techniques continue to underlie modern scientific method. Galen's discussion of the function of individual organs was vital in the formation of modern thinking on how internal organs relate to each other and are positioned in the body. Galen was also interested in the brain, theorizing that its function was related to the sense of smell.

Renaissance achievements

There was relatively little advancement of the concepts of the ancient Greeks and Romans until the start of the Renaissance—a time in European history that began in Italy at about the start of the 15th century. It was a period of intense intellectual questioning in all areas of scientific thought. The Italian Leonardo da Vinci (1452–1519), for example, created wax casts of the four ventricles in the brain to determine their volume and to monitor changes in the brain after death.

Ventricles
Each of the four connected fluid-filled cavities in the brain.

Anatomist
Someone who studies the bodily structure of living organisms.

In 1543 the Belgian anatomist Andreas Vesalius (1514–1564) challenged Galen's views of the brain. Vesalius performed dissections for his pupils. These dissections culminated in four anatomical charts that would influence the study of anatomy for more than 200 years after his death.

In 1573 the Italian physician Costanzo Varolio (1543–1575) became the first person to dissect the brain in its entirety, starting at the brain stem. In 1583 the German physician Felix Platter (1536–1614) dissected the human eye and realized that the eye only gathered light, dispelling the assumption that it also interpreted the information. Three years later the Italian physician Arcangelo Piccolomini (1525–1586) distinguished between two types of matter in the brain: the gray cortex and white matter. In 1587 the Italian physician Giulio Cesare Aranzi (1530–1589) clarified the nature of the brain's ventricles and identified the hippocampus deep within the brain.

Mind and matter

In 1623 the Italian scientist Galileo Galilei (1564–1642) proposed that science should only be concerned with "primary qualities"—those parts of the external world that could be measured or weighed. Galileo suggested that "secondary qualities," such as emotion, meaning, and value, did not fall into the realms of science. Throughout most of the 17th century, scientists concentrated their studies on the brain as a physical quantity. The science of neuroanatomy was born.

Systematic anatomy

Neuroanatomy owes more to English physician Thomas Willis (1621–1675) than to any other person. His book *Cerebri Anatome* (*Anatomy of the Brain*), a text on the anatomy of the central nervous system (brain and spinal cord), embraced the concept of blood circulation that the English physician William Harvey (1578–1657) had published in 1628. A part of the brain—a collection of arteries at the base of the brain called the circle of Willis—still bears his name. Willis understood that the circle was the interconnection of the major

---

Brain stem

The central part of a mammal's brain. It controls subconscious activities such as breathing, the sleep/wakefulness cycle, and heart rate.

Hippocampus

Part of the brain, thought to be the center of emotion, memory, and the autonomic nervous system.

Neuroanatomy

The study of the structure of the nervous system.

Arteries

Muscular-walled tubes conveying oxygenated blood from the heart to the rest of the body.

vessels supplying blood to the brain. He also suggested that cognitive functions, such as memory and vision, were located in specific places in the brain.

The brain and behavior

A major advance in the study of the physical workings of the brain came in 1791. The Italian scientist Luigi Galvani (1737–1798) showed that electricity existed within living things. The German physiologist Eduard Hitzig (1838–1907) was the first person to attempt stimulation of a living brain with an electrical current. He discovered that a small amount of current applied to the occipital lobes at the back of the head made his patients' eyes move to the left or the right. In 1870 Hitzig and his colleague Gustav Fritsch (1839–1927) stimulated the brains of live dogs and found that an electric current applied to specific parts of the outer layer made the dogs move specific body parts.

Simply observing people's behavior could also lead to great discoveries about the organization of the human brain. The British neurologist John Hughlings Jackson (1835–1911) noticed that the epileptic seizures of his wife followed a set pattern. The seizure would begin in one of her hands, move to the wrist, shoulder, and then to her face. Finally, it would affect

Cognitive
Relating to the gaining of knowledge and understanding through thought, experience, and the senses.

Curriculum Context

Students may be asked to describe how electrical stimulation in animal research can provide information about brain functions.

When Lobotomies Were Commonplace

At one time many patients underwent lobotomies—operations in which connections between the frontal lobes and the rest of the brain are severed. Widely used in the 1940s and 1950s, lobotomies are now performed only as a last resort in the treatment of severe, chronic depression. In the 1940s surgeons claimed a high success rate for prefrontal lobotomy operations in reducing aggressive behavior in violent patients. With the introduction of therapeutic drugs in the late 1950s, however, the practice was largely abandoned. It is now accepted that patients never recovered normal mental capacity. Some died prematurely and most are now in psychiatric care.

the leg on the same side of her body as the affected hand. Then the seizure would stop. Jackson came to believe that the seizures were caused by electric discharges in the brain. Further, the discharges started at one location within the brain and radiated outward, affecting other parts of the brain as they went. That suggested to Jackson that the brain is divided into parts, with each part related to a part of the body. Since the pattern of his wife's seizures never changed, Jackson theorized that the brain must be organized in a set pattern. These assumptions, formulated in 1865, were all proved correct.

Mapping the cortex

Wilder Graves Penfield (1891–1976) made several discoveries about the nature of the cortex in the 1950s. Penfield treated patients with severe epilepsy, many of whom reported that they felt a strange "aura" before having a seizure. Penfield realized that the feeling could be related to the exact areas in which the epilepsy originated.

Penfield anesthetized his patients but kept them conscious while he opened their skulls and attempted to find the origin of their epilepsy. Unexpectedly, stimulation of specific parts of the cortex led to specific associations for the patients. For example, if Penfield stimulated areas in the temporal lobes, he could provoke the memories of his patients. These memories were clearer than those recalled by usual means or were of events that had been forgotten. If Penfield stimulated the same area at different times, the same memory would be evoked.

Penfield also located the areas of nerves within the cortex that are activated by touch sensations in the skin of different parts of the body. Much more touch-related information is received from the face, lips, hands, and fingers than from other parts of the body.

Cortex

The outer layer of the brain that is concerned with consciousness.

Curriculum Context

Students may be asked to explain how touch sensory systems operate.

That is due to the presence of much higher concentrations of sensory receptors in the skin of these particular body parts. Areas such as the arms, torso, and legs have relatively few receptors. Penfield found that dense concentrations of receptors were connected to relatively large areas of cortex, while body areas with fewer receptors were served by smaller areas of cortex.

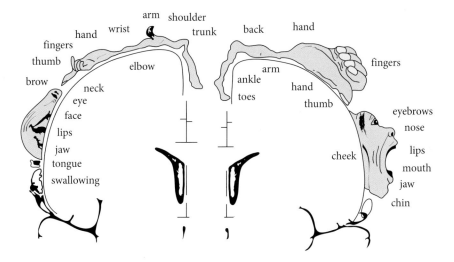

Penfield's map of the cortex shows the specific areas of the brain that are involved with the body's sense of touch. The areas of the body are enlarged in proportion to the amount of touch-related information that they convey to the brain.

Evolution and the brain

Many philosophers and scientists have tried to understand why the human brain has developed skills that far outstrip the brains of all other species. When the English naturalist Charles Darwin (1809–1882) published *On the Origin of Species* in 1859, he provided new and convincing answers to these questions.

The heart of Darwin's theory is that all living things evolved from a few common ancestors by a mechanism called natural selection. According to this theory, some organisms are better able to adapt to their environment and overcome pressures such as starvation, predation, and disease. These individuals are more likely to live longer and leave a greater number of offspring than other members of their species. The parents pass on the advantage to their offspring, and so the proportion of better-adapted individuals increases from one generation to the next.

Human evolution

Anthropologists believe that humans share a common ancestor with apes such as chimpanzees and gorillas. They point out that the fossilized remains of ancient humanlike beings and apes reveal many similarities.

The ancestors of modern humans probably began evolving separately from the ancestors of apes between 10 million and 5 million years ago. This period marks the beginning of the development of the hominids. The oldest-known hominids—the australopithecines, or australopiths for short—first appeared in Africa around 4 million years ago and died out somewhere between 2 million and 1 million years ago. The fossilized remains of australopith skulls suggest that the surface area of the cortex was large, although the brain was only one-third the size of our own.

The next step in human evolution came around 2.4 million years ago, again only in Africa, with the appearance of hominids from the genus *Homo*. The link between the australopiths and the earliest example, *Homo habilis*, has yet to be discovered, but fossil evidence indicates that *Homo habilis* had a larger brain and cortex surface area than the australopiths. They were the first hominids to make and use tools.

Homo erectus appears to have evolved from *Homo habilis* around 1.9 million years ago, again with a slightly larger brain and cortex surface area and an ability to light fires. *Homo erectus* was a successful

Anthropologists

Scientists who study human zoology, evolution, and culture.

Hominids

A group consisting of modern people and early humanlike ancestors.

Genus

A grouping of organisms that share common characteristics. Scientific names consist of two words: the genus name, followed by the species name.

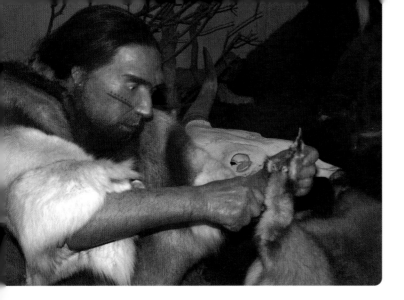

The Neanderthals appeared around 200,000 years ago. The brain size of a Neanderthal was similar to that of a modern human. Whether Neanderthals form the evolutionary link between *Homo erectus* and modern humans is still a matter of controversy.

species. Fossil evidence indicates that *Homo erectus* spread from Africa to colonize Asia and Europe.

Early forms of *Homo sapiens*, the direct ancestor of modern human beings, first appeared about 500,000 years ago. *Homo sapiens* had an even larger brain capacity than *Homo erectus*. The first modern humans, *Homo sapiens sapiens,* first appeared around 120,000 years ago. Around 80,000 years later that same species developed Cro-Magnon culture. Tools became more sophisticated, primitive cave artwork appeared, and agriculture set the stage for modern civilization.

Brain anatomy and intelligence

The area of the brain known as the brain stem appears to have changed very little from early in the evolutionary development of all mammals. Even reptiles, which developed much earlier than mammals, have a similar brain stem, with the same major nerve pathways. Brain-stem activities are crucial for survival. They include the regulation of breathing, heartbeat, and blood-sugar levels. These activities are considered to be reflex, or subconscious, actions.

Paul MacLean suggested that the human brain was three brains that had evolved in succession, one atop

Curriculum Context

Many curricula expect students to be able to summarize the function of the brain stem.

Curriculum Context

Understanding the way in which the human brain has evolved helps students understand the functions of the major brain regions.

Thalamus

The part of the brain whose role is to relay information from the body's senses to the cortex and to inform different parts of the brain what is going on in the body.

the other. At the base is the hindbrain, or "reptile brain," so-called because it contains all the structures needed for a reptile to survive. It consists of a small clump of cells atop the spine, to which the cerebellum—a clump of brain cells that control movement—is attached. Around the reptile brain is the second-level brain: the forebrain, or "old-mammalian brain." It contains structures that are developed in mammals but not very well developed in reptiles. Collectively known as the limbic system, these structures—the thalamus, amygdala, hippocampus, and hypothalamus—increase the range of mammalian behavior but are still largely concerned with basic functions such as reproduction and self-preservation. They also include some emotions. The "new mammalian brain" contains the most recently evolved parts of the mammalian nervous system, including the outer layer of the brain—the cerebral neocortex, or just cortex for short.

The Theory of Mind—Uniquely Human?

Fossil evidence and DNA analysis suggests that humans and nonhuman primates, such as chimpanzees and gorillas, share a common ancestor. However, many psychologists argue that humans are the only species with a theory of mind: Individuals understand that other individuals do not necessarily want or need the same things that they themselves do.

Recent research led by Brian Hare suggests that chimpanzees have at least some degree of a theory of mind. Chimpanzees are animals with a hierarchical social structure. So a dominant chimpanzee always eats first, followed by the subordinate members of its group. Hare placed two chimps in two cages separated by a central

cage in which he placed food. The subordinate chimpanzee could see all the food, but some of the food was hidden from the dominant chimpanzee. Changing the chimps' sightlines by moving the cages around, Hare discovered that the subordinate chimp would take any food that the dominant chimp could not see, as long as it could not be seen doing it. The subordinate chimp's behavior showed its awareness that the dominant chimp would want the food and indeed had its usual right to it. At the same time, it demonstrated an awareness of the other chimp's mind. Not only did the chimpanzee use its awareness of what the other chimpanzee could do, it also used the information to plan future decisions.

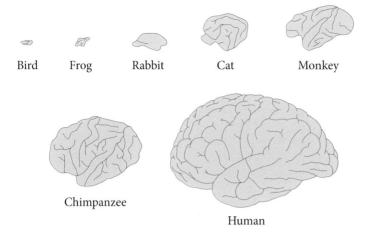

Bird   Frog   Rabbit   Cat   Monkey

Chimpanzee

Human

The cortex

The cortex is almost entirely exclusive to mammals. While all mammals may have areas of cortex in their brains, there is a great deal of variation between species in how much the cortex is folded into sulci (fissures) and gyri (ridges). Fissures and ridges greatly increase the total surface area of a cortex. Many scientists think that a greater degree of folding corresponds to an increased level of intelligence.

Superimposed systems

During the evolution of the human brain, new systems developed while old systems were still in use. Consequently the brain possesses more than one system to process information from certain senses. Where the human brain has two systems that perform the same task, the newer system always completes the task more efficiently than the older one.

The end of evolution?

Some scientists now argue that human evolution has reached its pinnacle. Other scientists argue that the future of human evolution depends on the brain continuing to develop an increased capacity to store and use knowledge.

The relative size of the brain in a human, a chimpanzee, a monkey, a cat, a rabbit, a frog, and a bird. Even if it is measured relative to the mass of the animal's body, the size of the brain does not prove to be an accurate way of determining general intelligence. Scientists now think that the degree of folding in the cerebral cortex is a better measure of intelligence.

Fissure

A long, narrow opening in the form of a crack or a groove.

Curriculum Context

Students should be able to link evolutionary brain development to challenges in the environment.

Biology of the Brain

The brain is an amazing organ. It holds our memories, dreams, fears, hopes, and every thought we have, both conscious and unconscious. Through the nervous system it controls activities of the body that we are not even aware are happening, as well as those we are aware of.

The human nervous system has two major divisions: The central nervous system (CNS), made up of the brain and spinal cord, and the peripheral nervous system.

Peripheral nervous system

The peripheral nervous system (PNS) sends information to and receives commands from the CNS. It comprises the spinal and cranial nerves, which connect the CNS to the rest of the body. The spinal nerves interact with the brain via the spinal cord. They link the CNS to the rest of the body. The cranial nerves interact directly with the brain and are largely concerned with the head, back, and shoulders. They connect the brain to the eyes, ears, and other parts of the head.

Autonomic and somatic systems

The PNS is itself divided into two parts, the autonomic nervous system and the somatic nervous system. The autonomic nervous system controls the automatic (unconscious or involuntary) internal body functions. The somatic nervous system controls the skeletal muscles, which are attached to the skeleton and govern voluntary (deliberate or conscious) movements. Neurons (nerve cells) send information via both systems. Afferent, or sensory, neurons carry information from the internal organs or from receptors in the eyes, ears, nose, tongue, and skin toward the CNS. Efferent, or motor, neurons carry information from the CNS to the internal organs in the autonomic system and to muscles in the somatic system.

Curriculum Context

Students should be able to identify the parts and subdivisions of the peripheral nervous system.

Curriculum Context

Students may find it useful to compare the functions of the autonomic and somatic nervous systems.

Cranial Nerves

There are 12 pairs of cranial nerves. Each cranial nerve includes both sensory and motor neurons, so they both receive information from and send information to the central nervous system. Unlike spinal nerves, cranial nerves link directly to the brain. They do not link via the spinal cord. In this illustration only one nerve of each pair is labeled.

- The olfactory nerves deal with smells.
- The optic nerves deal with vision.
- Three pairs of nerves (oculomotor, trochlear, and abducent) control movements of the eyes:
- The trigeminal nerves control jaw movements and sensation in the face.
- The facial nerves regulate facial expressions.
- The auditory nerves deal with sounds.
- The glossopharyngeal and hypoglossal nerves regulate the actions of tasting, chewing, and swallowing.
- The vagus nerves are concerned with breathing, blood circulation, and digestion.
- The spinal accessory nerves detect changes in muscles of the neck and back.

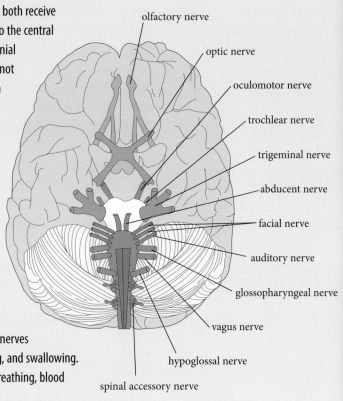

olfactory nerve
optic nerve
oculomotor nerve
trochlear nerve
trigeminal nerve
abducent nerve
facial nerve
auditory nerve
glossopharyngeal nerve
vagus nerve
hypoglossal nerve
spinal accessory nerve

The autonomic nervous system can be divided into two systems: the sympathetic and parasympathetic systems. Both conduct nerve impulses from the CNS to the body's internal organs. Together the sympathetic and parasympathetic nerves control how much energy each body organ should have and when each should have it. Levels of nerve activity in each of the two systems and the interaction between them decide the outcome for each organ. Sympathetic nerves stimulate activity, while parasympathetic nerves reduce activity.

Pelvis

The large bony structure near the base of the spine to which the legs are connected: the hipbone forms the main part of the pelvis.

Membranes

Thin, pliable sheets that act as boundaries or partitions in the body.

Curriculum Context

Many curricula expect students to summarize the functions of the major brain regions.

Central nervous system

The spinal cord is a length of nerve tissue that runs from the hindbrain to the pelvis; it is protected by the vertebrae (interconnecting bones) of the spine, or backbone. A cross section of the spinal cord shows a gray mass surrounded by white tissue. The gray matter contains a high density of nerve cell bodies that connect directly to neurons joining the spinal cord from elsewhere in the body. The white matter consists of neurons that send information up and down the spinal cord. A layer of myelin, a fatty substance, covers the white matter.

The meninges

The spinal cord and the brain are protected by three membranes called meninges. The outer membrane is a tough covering called the dura mater. Inside the dura mater is the arachnoid mater, which has a spongy consistency. Below this is the subarachnoid space, which houses blood vessels. Sticking to the surface of the nervous tissues of the brain and spinal cord is the delicate pia mater layer, which provides cushioning.

Cerebrospinal fluid

The brain and spinal cord are also protected by a liquid called cerebrospinal fluid which fills the subarachnoid space of the brain and spinal cord, and the hollow core, or central canal, of the spinal cord. Both spinal cord and brain are virtually suspended in this fluid. This cushions them from impacts caused by movements of the body.

Brain divisions

The brain has three distinct regions: the hindbrain, the midbrain, and the forebrain. Anatomists divide them into five parts, each of which owes its existence to an evolutionary advance from other animals.

Hindbrain 1: the myelencephalon

The region of the hindbrain called the myelencephalon is also known as the medulla oblongata. The

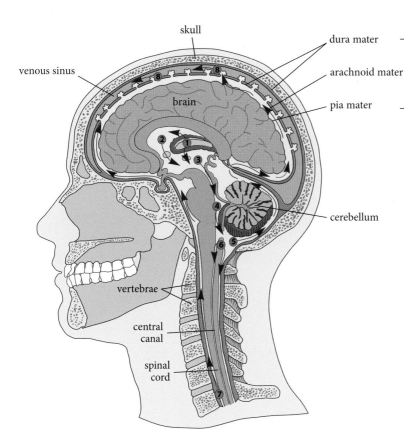

skull

venous sinus

brain

dura mater

arachnoid mater

pia mater

cerebellum

vertebrae

central canal

spinal cord

Diagram of a skull and brain sliced in half, showing the ventricles (chambers). Cerebrospinal fluid is produced by the linings (1) of all the ventricles. The fluid flows from the lateral ventricles (2) to the third (3) and fourth (4) ventricles. From the fourth ventricle the fluid flows up the rear of the brain (5) along the subarachnoid space. Fluid flows down the spinal cord along the central canal and the rear subarachnoid space (6). The fluid flows up the front of the spinal cord (7). After circulating, the fluid is reabsorbed into the blood via projections of the arachnoid mater (8) that connect to a blood vessel called the venous sinus.

myelencephalon transmits information from other parts of the brain to the spinal cord, from where it travels to the rest of the body. Within the myelencephalon is a structure named the reticular formation, which is heavily involved in almost all of our autonomic nervous system activities, including sleeping and respiratory (breathing) reflexes. It also has a role in cognitive (information-processing) activities such as the focusing of attention and the direction of movement.

Hindbrain 2: the metencephalon
The metencephalon is the second half of the hindbrain. It is divided into two main parts: the pons and the cerebellum. The pons is a bulge on the surface of the brain stem that houses that part of the reticular formation not contained in the myelencephalon. Some cranial nerves exit the pons.

The cerebellum is a large structure at the back of the brain stem. Its appearance is a bit like that of a cauliflower or broccoli. Its main function is related to motor activity, and it is vital to the sensorimotor system—the interaction of sense receptors and muscular responses.

Midbrain: the mesencephalon

The midbrain, or mesencephalon, is covered by a layer of tissue called the tectum. On the roof of the midbrain the tectum forms two pairs of lumps called the inferior colliculi and the superior colliculi. The inferior colliculi are involved in processing information from the ears, while the superior colliculi process information from the eyes. The midbrain also contains the cerebral aqueduct, which connects the third and the fourth ventricles. The cerebral aqueduct is surrounded by the periaqueductal gray, which has a pain-reducing role similar to that of opiate drugs. Also within the midbrain are areas called the substantia nigra and the red nucleus, which are vital to the sensorimotor system.

Forebrain 1: the diencephalon

The diencephalon and the telencephalon are the two parts of the forebrain. The diencephalon includes the thalamus and the hypothalamus.

The thalamus sits on the top of the brain stem and is shaped into two lobes connected by the massa intermedia, a band of gray tissue. The thalamus is often regarded as a relay station between the senses and the cortex (the outer layer of the brain). The thalamus processes raw data and sends the information to the correct areas of the cortex.

The hypothalamus plays a vital part in many behaviors and activities of the body, including emotional states, and influences some of them by controlling the release of hormones from the pituitary gland, which is

Motor activity

Control of the muscles.

Opiate drugs

Drugs derived from opium that cause drowsiness or dull the senses.

Hormones

Substances released into the bloodstream to regulate the behavior of specific cells or tissues.

directly connected to the hypothalamus. The pituitary gland is sometimes called the master gland because its function is to compel other glands to release hormones. The pituitary gland is very important for sexual functions; among other things, it triggers the menstrual period in women.

The optic chiasm—part of the diencephalon—is where optic nerves (from the eyes) join together. From the optic chiasm the nerves run into the brain. The optic chiasm forms an **X** since some nerves cross from each of the eyes to parts of the brain on the opposite side of the head. The left visual field (range of vision) from both eyes is sent to the right side of the brain, while information from the right visual field is sent to the left side of the brain.

Locations of the five main regions of the brain.

myelencephalon

metencephalon

mesencephalon

diencephalon

telencephalon

Forebrain 2: the telencephalon

The telencephalon includes the two cerebral hemispheres and their outer layer, or cortex. It is the area of the brain where much information is received, processed, and stored, and where voluntary movements are initiated. Functions such as learning, memory, language comprehension, and problem solving are all housed in the telencephalon.

Cerebral cortex

The cortex is a wrinkly layer of tissue that covers the outside of the cerebral hemispheres. The wrinkles increase the amount of cortex that can fit within the skull. The large wrinkles are known as fissures, while smaller wrinkles are referred to as sulci. Gyri are the ridges between the wrinkles. The longitudinal fissure divides the two hemispheres of the brain. Bundles of nerve cells called commissures provide communication between the hemispheres. Each hemisphere has a

Hemisphere
One of the two halves—left and right—of the brain.

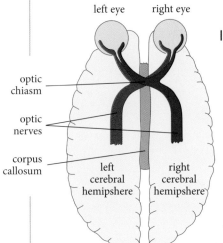

left eye   right eye

optic
chiasm

optic
nerves

corpus
callosum

left
cerebral
hemipshere

right
cerebral
hemipshere

The two hemispheres of the human brain are cross-wired in many ways. This diagram shows how optic nerves cross to form the X-shaped optic chiasm. The corpus callosum is a thick bundle of nerve tissue that links the two hemispheres.

Nerves that collect data from the right field of vision.

Nerves that collect data from the left field of vision.

lateral fissure, and the central fissure increases the size of the cortex. The precentral gyrus contains detailed information on the layout of the body and is related to muscle-activating activities. The postcentral gyrus is largely related to the body's sensory receptor system.

Anatomists use the fissures to define the four main lobes of each cerebral hemisphere. They are the frontal lobe, the temporal lobe, the parietal lobe, and the occipital lobe. In evolutionary terms the frontal lobes are the most recent addition to the human brain and contain areas involved in people's most complex cognitive functions and behaviors.

The parietal lobes process spatial information in advanced ways, such as the creation of mental images and the recognition of people's faces. The parietal lobes also have some relationship with the proprioceptive system, which senses movement in the body's tissues.

The main function of the occipital lobes is to process visual information. The optic nerve ends in this area, and the occipital lobes sort the information it carries into color, shape, and the identity of individual objects.

The temporal lobes receive information associated with hearing and the sense of balance from the thalamus and the cranial nerves. Wernicke's area, which is vital for language comprehension, resides in the left temporal lobe in many people. The transfer of short-term memories to long-term memory is also related to temporal lobe function.

Below the cortex much of the cerebral hemispheres is taken up by nerve connections between regions of the cortex. This area is termed the limbic system which motivates and links areas of the diencephalon and the telencephalon. Behaviors such as eating, fighting, escaping, and sexual arousal are all regulated by the limbic system.

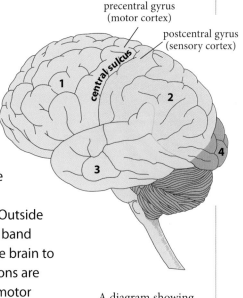

precentral gyrus
(motor cortex)

postcentral gyrus
(sensory cortex)

central sulcus

1

2

4

3

A diagram showing the four main lobes of the brain:

1. Frontal lobe
2. Parietal lobe
3. Temporal lobe
4. Occipital lobe

Neurons

In the human nervous system there are two main types of cells: neurons and glial cells. Neurons (nerve cells) may communicate with each other on an individual basis or as networked collections of millions or billions. Outside the central nervous system (CNS), nerve cells band together to form cablelike nerves that link the brain to the rest of the body via the spinal cord. Neurons are classified by function into three main types: motor neurons, sensory neurons, and interneurons.

Motor neurons carry messages from the CNS to muscles and glands. They trigger movements, deliberate or otherwise, and the release of hormones. A typical motor neuron looks like a tree, with a root system, a trunk, and a system of branches. The "roots" are referred to as dendrites. At the center of the "root system" lies the soma, or cell body. The "trunk" of the neuron is called the axon. The axon is covered by an insulating myelin sheath which speeds up the transmission of electricity from one neuron to another. The "branches" of the axon are at the opposite end from the dendrites, and each branch ends in a terminal button. The buttons connect with nearby neurons across a junction called the synapse. Each root and branch of the neuron is linked via synapses to the dendrites of many other neurons or to other tissues.

Myelin

A mixture of proteins and phospholipids that forms a whitish insulation around many nerve fibers.

Sensory neurons send nerve impulses from the eyes, ears, nose, tongue, and receptors in the body, organs, and skin to the CNS. Individual sensory neurons belong to certain sensory systems. Interneurons exist only in the CNS. A single interneuron connects many nerve cells to many other neurons and interneurons.

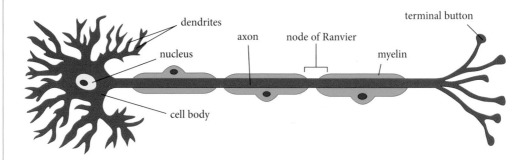

The main parts of a motor neuron. The nucleus is the cell's control center. The axon is the longest extension of the cell body. The axons of thousands of neurons make up the cablelike nerves of the peripheral nervous system. Dendrites are shorter extensions of the cell body. All extensions of a neuron's body, axons and dendrites, are called processes.

Glial cells

The CNS also contains glia, or glial cells. Glia support the neurons in their functions. They are essential for the formation of myelin sheaths around axons. Glia also clean neurons by flushing out old material, and they take the place of any neurons that die. They also supply the neurons with nutrients.

The nerve impulse

To perform their varied and complex tasks, neurons have to communicate with each other: electrically, via the nerve impulse (or action potential), and chemically using neurotransmitters. The synapse is the junction at which neurons communicate with each other as well as with muscles and glands. A synapse includes a synaptic cleft, or gap between the communicating cells; it also includes the terminal button sending the signal and the part of the dendrite receiving the impulse. The nerve impulse travels from the cell body, down the axon and to the terminal buttons.

Bags of chemicals in solution

All cells are like bags of chemicals in solution. The cell membrane encloses the cell and controls the flow of substances between the outside and the inside of the cell. The solution inside the membrane is known as intracellular fluid. Outside and between all the cells of the brain is the extracellular space, which is filled with extracellular fluid. Many vital chemicals are dissolved in these fluids. The most important are the concentrations of positively charged ions of sodium and potassium.

Ions

Atoms that have either a positive or a negative electrical charge. Sodium and potassium ions both have positive charges.

Resting potential

When the cell is not activated by a stimulus, the membrane stays in its resting state (or resting potential). The nerve cell constantly pumps sodium ions out of the cell and potassium ions into the cell. Both trickle back across the cell membrane, but at different rates. The result is a greater concentration of positive ions on the outside of the cell, which gives the inside of the cell a very small negative charge.

Action potential

A nerve impulse, or action potential, occurs when a neuron is stimulated to fire by neurotransmitters. Channels in the stimulated section of the membrane open up, and sodium ions flood into the cell, giving that section a sudden positive charge. As the difference in charge between the inside and the outside of the cell is reduced, potassium channels open up briefly. They allow potassium ions to flood out of the cell, so the interior is once again negative. By this time, however, the incoming sodium ions have triggered more sodium channels to open up in adjacent parts of the cell membrane and the whole process is repeated. The charge travels down the cell body and axon until it reaches the terminal buttons.

Motor and sensory neurons remain inactive unless stimulated by other neurons into firing a nerve impulse. Many other neurons in the CNS produce action potentials continuously, or at regular or irregular intervals.

Neurotransmitters

A nerve impulse has to get the message across the synapse using neurotransmitters. Inside the terminal buttons, tiny vesicles contain miniorgans that make neurotransmitters from chemicals inside the cell. When a nerve impulse reaches the membrane of a terminal button (presynaptic membrane) it causes some of the vesicles to fuse with the cell wall and spill molecules of

Curriculum Context

Curricula may ask students to discuss how internal and external stimuli initiate the communication process in the neuron.

Vesicles

Small fluid-filled cavities.

neurotransmitters into the synaptic cleft. Some molecules diffuse to the other side of the synapse and attach to receptors (special binding sites) in the membrane of the next neuron (called the postsynaptic membrane). Alternatively, the neurotransmitter may be taken up by the same neuron that discharged it.

Types of neurotransmitters

There are four main classes of known neurotransmitters, but more must exist since the brain performs functions that cannot be explained by only these four classes.

Amino acid neurotransmitters play a major role in most rapid changes in the synapses between neurons that lie close together.

Monoamine neurotransmitters are produced from a single amino acid. There are four main monoamine types. Dopamine is involved in movement, attention, and learning. It is used to make norepinephrine and epinephrine, which are involved in the regulation of alertness and the ability to respond rapidly to a threat. Serotonin plays a part in sleep and arousal, sensitivity to pain, and the control of appetite and mood.

Acetylcholine neurotransmitters are important at junctions between muscle cells and motor neurons, and make muscles contract. They also occur at synapses in the autonomic nervous system and are involved in memory function.

Neuropeptides

One important group of neurotransmitters is the neuropeptides (or peptides), which consist of chains of amino acid molecules. Many neuropeptides occur as hormones in other parts of the body. Those peptides are released by the endocrine glands but it appears that some peptides are produced by neurons to use as neurotransmitters.

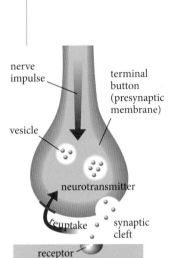

nerve impulse

terminal button (presynaptic membrane)

vesicle

neurotransmitter

reuptake

synaptic cleft

receptor

postsynaptic membrane

When a nerve impulse reaches the terminal button of a neuron, vesicles containing neurotransmitters fuse with the cell wall and release their contents into the synaptic cleft (gap between two communicating cells). The neurotransmitters bind to receptor sites on the postsynaptic membrane (of the nearby cell). Some are reabsorbed by the same cell that released them. This is termed reuptake.

Released peptides have a much more wide-reaching effect than other neurotransmitters, which act only locally. Peptides travel through the extracellular fluid into the brain's ventricles and the bloodstream. They can bind to cells that are in entirely different nerve systems from the releasing cell and can travel over the entire brain to find a suitable binding site. When a peptide eventually binds to a neuronal membrane, it causes a gradual change in the neuron that is triggered by second messengers (molecules formed by the peptide from chemicals in the cell membrane).

Neurotransmitter functions

Peptide neurotransmitters seem to either increase or decrease the sensitivity of a large number of neurons to the effects of other neurotransmitters, which appear to send short-lived messages to nearby postsynaptic receptors that act either to excite or inhibit formation of nerve impulses in the neuron.

A neurotransmitter can only excite or inhibit electrical activity in a neuron when it binds to the right type of receptor on the postsynaptic membrane. A transmitter deposited in the synapse will not be accepted by the postsynaptic membrane of the nearest dendrite if it has no receptors for that type of neurotransmitter.

Curriculum Context

Students can usefully contrast excitatory and inhibitory transmission of nerve impulses.

Prozac

The antidepressant drug Prozac (fluoxetine) first went on sale in the United States in 1987.

Research had indicated that low levels of serotonin are associated with sleeplessness and irritation, and that depression is relieved by maintaining normal serotonin levels. Prozac is a selective serotonin reuptake inhibitor (SSRI): It decreases reuptake by the presynaptic cell of a specific type of serotonin from the synapse. Levels of serotonin in the synaptic cleft therefore remain high. Reuptake of serotonin is performed by molecular pumps in the presynaptic membrane, and Prozac finds them and blocks them with its own molecules. Prozac also inhibits enzyme activity that breaks down serotonin in the synaptic cleft.

The Mind

Our perceptions of the world depend on the way in which physical stimuli operate on our bodies and generate thoughts, feelings, and consciousness. Conversely, our thoughts and desires clearly operate on our bodies and affect our actions. How can a physical object such as the brain operate on an intangible and invisible entity such as the mind?

Before psychology developed in the late 19th century, the answers to these questions lay in the realms of philosophy. The Greek philosopher Plato (c.428–348 B.C.) was perhaps the first person to put forward a theory on the nature of the mind. Plato argued that the mind was a nonphysical entity. He used the Greek word *psyche*, meaning "soul," to describe this invisible substance. He believed that it was separate and distinct from the rest of the body—the physical substance. Philosophers call Plato's theory of mind-and-body separation "dualism."

Curriculum Context

Students may be interested in exploring the influence of Plato's and Aristotle's ideas on philosophy up to the European Renaissance.

Aristotle (384–322 B.C.), another Greek philosopher, disagreed with Plato's theory. Aristotle thought that the mental substance ("form") and physical substance ("matter") were connected. Aristotle believed that every living thing was a combination of matter and form—each dependent on the other.

Later the ideas of Plato and Aristotle were taken up by the philosophers of a period in history called the Scholastic era. In addition the Scholastic philosophers believed that our ability to form ideas was a gift given by God. St. Augustine (A.D. 354–430) named this gift "illumination." The Scholastic idea of the nature of the mind continued to be popular well into the Middle Ages.

The Cartesian model
The French mathematician and philosopher René Descartes (1596–1650) decided to build a completely

new system of philosophy based on his own foundations. Descartes decided to doubt everything. Desperately, he looked for something that would be impossible to question. The revelation came when Descartes realized the one fact that he could not deny: the fact that he was doubting. Only one thing cannot be doubted: doubt itself. His discovery is summed up in the famous philosophical argument "I think, therefore I am." Once Descartes felt safe that he existed, he felt he could also be sure that the world around him existed. He then began to look for differences between himself and the natural world, which he believed was shaped by physical laws. But he could not apply the same rules to his mind. So, like Plato, Descartes believed in dualism but that mind and body could interact, forming a "union" that resulted in a human being.

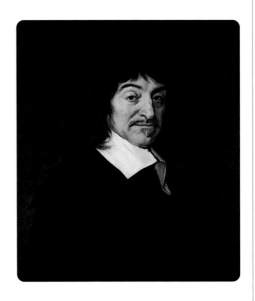

René Descartes tried to synthesize philosophy and mathematics or, as he put it, "bridge the gulf between the domain of natural science and the soul." He believed that mental operations could be represented by abstract symbols "in the same system as the perceptual states that produced them" and used symbols from algebra to explain his theory of mental representation.

Perspectives post-Descartes

Descartes's work prompted many philosophers to attempt to solve the "mind-body problem." The English empiricist philosopher John Locke (1632–1704) moved the debate into the psychological realm of experience. Locke did not think that the physical or the mental was really fundamental. The reality was somewhere neutral between them. Locke described the mind as a "blank slate" and argued that people gained knowledge through experience. Sensory experience, or sensation, provided one kind of experience. The other, which Locke called reflection, was the mind's combination and comparison of various sensory impressions.

Locke went on to argue that, while we cannot prove that the material world exists, our senses give us evidence affording all the certainty that we need. He regarded it as impossible for humans to have any understanding of the relation between mind and body. All the perceptions of one's own body, as of the rest of the physical world, are ideas in the mind.

Curriculum Context

Students can usefully compare Locke's and Hume's views on how we accumulate knowledge.

Scotsman David Hume (1711–1776) developed a theory of knowledge based on scientific principles. Like Locke, Hume thought that the mind does not create ideas but forms them from the senses. Hume went on to define knowledge as either "relations of matter" or "matters of fact." Ideas are simply related meanings, for example, that movement consists of the relationship between space and time. Matters of fact must be accepted for what they are, for example, that grass is green and that fire is hot.

Theory of Mind

The question of what makes us uniquely human has been hotly debated since the dawn of recorded history. What is it that sets us apart from other animals? Maybe it is because we can think about thinking, as well as think about what other people are thinking, and act on the conclusions reached. That is what is generally referred to as theory of mind (TOM). TOM includes the capacity for self-reflection, the ability to articulate understanding of one's own thoughts and knowledge, together with some degree of insight into what others know and think.

Some investigations of the development of mind have been based on the idea that when children begin to have a capacity for deception, it is because they have begun to realize that not everyone knows what they know. In other words, they have made the discovery that sometimes they have unique knowledge that others do not have. This kind of development usually occurs between the ages of three and five years.

In many ways chimpanzees are very similar to humans—they are highly intelligent and can communicate with each other and with us. Fossil evidence and the analysis of DNA suggest that we share a common ancestor with chimps. Physically, a chimp's brain is very similar to ours, too. So do chimps possess TOM? Recent evidence suggests that they do. Deception has been observed in many chimp behaviors. For example, subordinate males have been known to attempt "sneaky" matings with females out of sight of the alpha (dominant) male. Chimps have also been known to make false alarm calls to scare the troop away from a tree laden with fruit so that they can eat it all themselves.

Hume was troubled by the concept of causality. He believed that the knowledge of the relationship between matters of fact, such as a fire (cause) being hot (effect), result from an internal association of the two ideas "fire" and "hot." The knowledge of causality comes from the accumulation of subjective experiences. The implication of this idea is that cause-and-effect relationships are based on subjectivity. Scientists try to be objective, but since they rely on observing causal relationships, science itself is based on subjectivity. So there can be no rational, scientific theory of how we accumulate knowledge.

Immanuel Kant

In the 18th century the German philosopher Immanuel Kant (1724–1804) attempted to combine the theories of the empiricists Locke and Hume with those of Descartes and other rationalist philosophers. Unlike the empiricists, who state that all knowledge is based on the accumulation of sensory experiences, rationalists believe that knowledge can be gained just by thinking and reasoning.

The problem of knowledge, as Kant viewed it, was how to link sensory experiences with innate knowledge, that is, knowledge we all have from birth. His starting point was to distinguish between analytic and synthetic judgments. Analytic judgments are ones in which the truth of such a judgment can be known by analyzing the subject. A synthetic judgment is one in which the truth of a statement cannot be known through analyzing the subject.

Kant also distinguished two ways in which humans can accumulate knowledge. Something is known "a priori" if it cannot be derived from or tested by any sensory experiences. Something is known "a posteriori" if it can be derived from or tested by experience.

Causality
The cause and effect in any relationship.

Subjective
Influenced by personal feelings or opinions.

Empiricist
Someone who believes that knowledge is based on observation or experience rather than on theory or logic.

Rationalist
Believing that opinions and actions should be based on reason or logic.

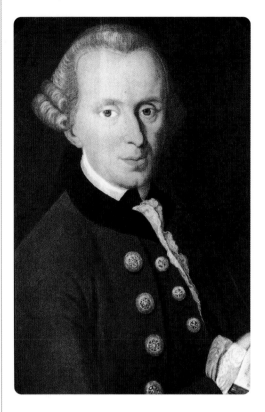

Immanuel Kant called his theory the "Copernican Revolution" of philosophy. Just as Nicolaus Copernicus (1473–1543) reversed the way scientists viewed the relationship between the Earth and the Sun, so Kant reversed the way that philosophers viewed the relationship between the world of experience and the world of the mind.

Kant called the innate contribution of the mind a "category" and listed four different categories by which the contents of experience are ordered. The categories are quantity (how much of something), quality (the types of things), relation (how things interact), and modality (what things can be). We apply them to our everyday experiences to make sense of the world. The innate contribution of the mind gives meaning to our experiences. The mind is not shaped by the world of experience; rather the world of experience is shaped by the patterns set by the mind.

Whether things really are the way they appear to us is something we can never know because all our knowledge is prestructured by the mind. This is the basis for Kant's famous distinction between the unknowable noumenon ("thing-in-itself") and the phenomenon ("thing-as-it-appears").

A science of mind

The study of the mind remained the province of philosophical debate until the end of the 19th century. Then three major developments laid the foundations for the scientific study of the mind.

The first was made by Franz Brentano (1838–1917). In 1874 Brentano tried to establish a systematic study of psychology that would form the basis of a science of the mind. Brentano revived the Scholastic philosophical theory of intentionality. The concept of intentionality enables philosophers to deal with the problems of dualism by relating what appears in the mind to the real object. Some dualist philosophers think that an experienced and remembered object can exist in our consciousness even though the real object exists outside the mind. Brentano's theory of intentionality avoided the question of whether consciousness exists. We direct our consciousness onto the object and recognize it. The word "intentionality" comes from the Latin *intendo*, meaning "to aim at or point toward." The only problems Brentano faced were how the object comes to have a meaning for our consciousness and how our mind relates to the object.

The second breakthrough was the establishment of psychology as a distinct scientific discipline in the 19th century. The German physiologist and psychologist Wilhelm Wundt opened the first psychology laboratory at the University of Leipzig, Germany, in 1879. Wundt and his colleagues were trying to study the mind using a process called "introspection"—a method in which people observe and analyze their own thoughts, feelings, and mental images. The subjects recorded their introspections under controlled conditions, and Wundt used the same physical surroundings and the same stimuli for each experiment.

The last major breakthrough in the development of a science of the mind was made by the American philosopher and psychologist William James (1842–1910). James published his *Principles of Psychology* in 1890, which assimilated mental science into a purely biological discipline and treated thinking and knowledge as tools in the struggle to survive. At the same time, James made the fullest use of principles of psychophysics.

Seeds of doubt
Within a few decades the experimental methods of Wundt became overshadowed by the behaviorist approach. According to behaviorists such as the

The Evolution of a Science

Psychology first arrived as a fully fledged science in 1879, when Wilhelm Wundt set up a laboratory designed to explore systematically the operation of perception. This earliest school of psychology has become known as structuralism. It tried to identify and define the building blocks of mental structures such as the formation of concepts, planning, and thinking. Structuralists believed that these structures were the basis of consciousness. Wundt claimed to have objectively identified the two main components of consciousness: sensations (hearing, smell, taste, touch, and vision) and feelings (such as anger, fear, and love). One problem with these findings was that the primary research technique used to reach these conclusions was introspection. It requires people to think about what they think and do, and to report their findings. For example, subjects might be given several pieces of information to memorize or a problem to solve; they are then asked to describe what went through their minds while they were performing these tasks. People will report only those processes of which they are aware. In addition, any description of what happened, no matter how detailed or accurate, is not a description of how it happened. Moreover, the results of such experiments produce subjective results based on the personal experience of the subject. Thus theories based on introspection fell out of fashion.

Curriculum Context

Students should be able to explain behaviorist objections to the research technique of introspection.

American psychologist John B. Watson (1878–1958), psychologists could learn more about the workings of the mind by studying the relationship between observable stimuli and the consequent behavioral responses. Extreme versions of behaviorism denied the existence of the mind. Most behaviorists thought that introspection was flawed as a method of analysis. If people report their experiences after the introspection, they rely on memory, which experiments have shown can be inaccurate. Second, people do not have access to the inner workings of their mental processes and so cannot be expected to account for them. Third, introspection yields subjective results—opinionated thoughts as opposed to unbiased, objective information.

Cognitive science

In the 1950s a new field of study called cognitive science revolutionized psychology. Cognitive science developed from quite disparate fields of study. In 1956 a study published by George A. Miller (born 1920) showed that the capacity of human thought is limited. Miller suggested that most people can store only seven plus or minus two pieces of information in short-term memory and demonstrated a way of improving the capacity of short-term memory by storing chunks of information. Miller's study went some way to explain the mechanisms by which the mind stores information in the form of coded, mental representations.

The second major influence on the cognitive science revolution was made by the American linguist Noam Chomsky (born 1928). In 1959 he published a study that showed that language was much more complex than anyone had previously believed. Language could not be a learned habit, as behaviorists thought. Chomsky viewed language as a way to express ideas and said that these ideas are expressed according to mental grammar in the form of rules.

Linguist
Someone who studies languages and their structure.

Another important driving force was the invention of the first computing machines in the late 1940s. Soon after, pioneers in cognitive science constructed computer models of the mind and attempted to build computers with artificial intelligence.

Neuroscience

As cognitive science brings about new understanding about the mind, so neuroscience brings new understanding about the workings of the brain. Neuroscientists base their observations on empirical research. For example, they insert electrodes into the brain to record the activity of individual neurons. The neuroscientist then tries to work out how the billions of connected neurons that form our brains produce such a complex set of cognitive abilities. In addition, a new breed of cognitive psychologists, called cognitive

Neuroscience
The study of the structure and function of the brain.

Electrodes
The conductors through which electricity enters or leaves an object.

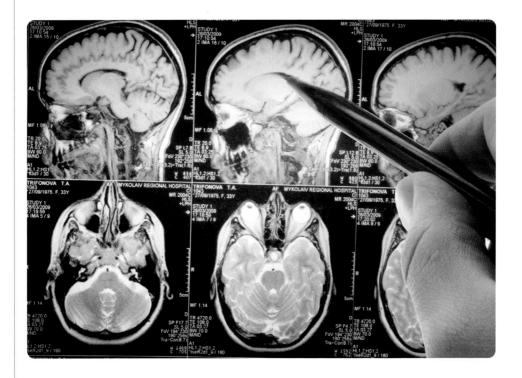

Neuroscientists use noninvasive brain-imaging technologies, such as magnetic resonance imaging (MRI) and positron emission tomography (PET) scanning equipment, to record brain activity while people perform various mental tasks. The images produced by these scans have identified areas of the brain that are involved in specific tasks, such as mental imagery and language processing.

neuropsychologists, gather data by observing the disabilities of people whose brains have been damaged.

A new philosophy

Very few modern philosophers perform experiments or construct computer models of the mind to formulate their theories. They deal with general issues such as the relation of the mind and body and try to explain the concepts derived by cognitive scientists. In turn, the work of cognitive scientists can help improve philosophical approaches.

Very few philosophers now subscribe to Descartes's dualist view. They argue that the mind must be viewed as some part of the physical world. Much of the recent philosophical debate aims to establish the laws that govern the mind. There are a number of theories that form a broad school of philosophy called materialism.

Identity theory

One of these theories, identity theory, or reductive materialism, is a simple idea. Proponents believe that mental states are identical, or related, to neural pathways in the brain. As more of these pathways are mapped, we may soon be able to denote mental processes like "desiring" with the activity of neurons (nerve cells) in one section of a particular area of the brain. Identity theory has failed to convince most philosophers and psychologists. The main problem has been trying to match various mental activities to particular neurons in the brain.

Functionalism

The criticisms leveled against identity theory have led to the development of another theory called functionalism. Functionalists believe that behavior is a result of a collection of mental processes and try to explain mental processes in terms of cause-and-effect relationships, which they call functions. Functionalists try to recognize the functions that produce certain behaviors and what those behaviors will be. They also allow for multiple meanings for different mental processes, so they do not think that behaviors can be pinpointed to specific areas of neural activity.

Eliminative materialism

In its most extreme view, eliminative materialism advocates the elimination of psychological categories, such as attention and memory, in favor of a scientific explanation at the neurobiological level. This theory is known as reductionism and holds that neuroscience can provide an explanation for all mental events. So psychology can be reduced to neuroscience and eventually to chemistry and physics.

Philosopher Patricia Churchland believes that the mind should be investigated through multiple levels of research—molecular, cellular, functional, behavioral, systemwide, and brainwide—all at the same time. Churchland believes that the results of each approach should be used to inform the others and thus improve our overall understanding of the mind.

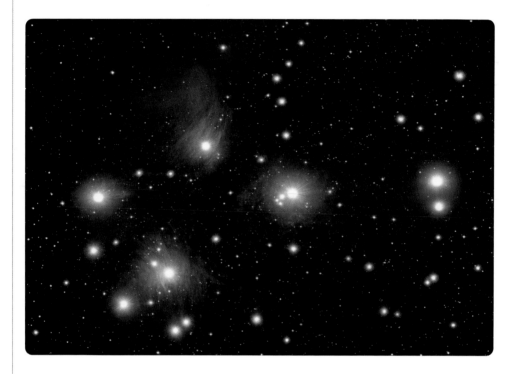

The light emitted by stars takes so long to reach Earth that we are seeing them not as they are now but as they used to be, often millions of years ago. This is analogous to the backward referral hypothesis of Benjamin Libet, which suggests that because of the time lapse between the receipt of a stimulus and its interpretation by our brains, we are living a fraction of a second in the past.

Backward referral hypothesis
In the 1990s, Benjamin Libet came to the conclusion that we are living in the past. Not very far in the past, only about half a second; but it takes that much time for us to become consciously aware of our perceptions. By the time we become aware of stimuli and decide in our mind how to respond to them, our brain has often

already initiated a possible response. These experiments formed the basis of his "backward referral hypothesis." Fortunately, backward referral is not so delayed that we act without thinking. Awareness occurs so quickly that we have time to override any inappropriately triggered response. Libet believes that this ability to detect and correct instinctive misjudgments is the basis of free will.

The functions of the mind

When we consider the activities of the mind, it seems we need to consider a whole host of mental processes. To begin with, let us look at how the brain takes in information from external stimuli so that we can interact with the world—in other words, the workings of sensation and perception.

How can we listen to a song on the radio, watch a football game on television, understand what a friend is saying to us on the phone—and, indeed, often perform more than one of these activities at the same time? When we consider the complexity of such processes, it is amazing that we can take up so much information. Somehow we synthesize all this seemingly disparate information to form integrated perceptions, so that we can act, react, and survive.

To understand how these perceptional functions work, it is useful to compare them with situations in which they have become a problem. Take the case of P. T., a man who, after sustaining brain damage, had particular difficulty in recognizing objects and people around him. The woman who served him his breakfast every morning was a complete stranger. He had no trouble seeing her. He could even describe her actions as she walked across the kitchen. He simply failed to recognize her—until she spoke. On hearing her voice he would suddenly realize that it was his wife. P. T. suffered from a condition known as visual agnosia.

Agnosia

The inability to recognize sensations.

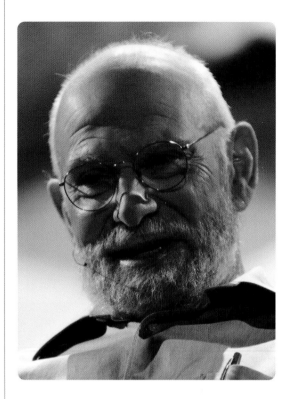

P. T. had normal vision but his brain could not make sense of it all. This was not a disorder of sensation; it was a disorder of perception. In visual agnosia the single stimulus of sight is insufficient to trigger recognition, but the combination of sight with other stimuli may enable sufferers to recognize previously unperceived wholes. Other agnosias—auditory (inability to recognize familiar sounds) and tactile (inability to recognize familiar objects through touch)—may be relieved by supplying the sufferer with visual information.

The British neurologist Oliver Sacks (born 1933) described a case of visual agnosia in which a man could not tell the difference between his wife's face and his own hat until he heard her voice.

Curriculum Context

It may be useful to design an experiment that illustrates the difference between selective attention and divided attention.

Attention and the mind

To act, react, and survive in the world, we need to know how to select and recognize what we perceive. The ability to do these things is known as "attention," but what exactly is it?

Certainly we can choose what to pay attention to. We have to, or we would be overwhelmed by information. We have probably all experienced some variation of this phenomenon—perhaps in a library while studying. You may be concentrating on a particularly confusing text. Perhaps you are struggling because you are simultaneously aware of friends nearby talking about the day's baseball game. So you must choose which input to respond to. You cannot follow both trains of thought. You may decide to tune out the baseball game discussion and concentrate on the text in front of you. But are you completely cut off from your friends' conversation? Research shows that you are not. You have merely decided not to select various pieces of information that have entered your brain through your ears. If the other people suddenly start talking about the thing you particularly want to know—in this case the score—you will suddenly tune out of your text and in to their conversation.

Voluntary and reflexive attention

The problem described above is an example of what is called voluntary attention. The other type of attention is reflexive attention: If we are working and the phone rings, we are immediately and involuntarily distracted from our work to listen to the sound. By and large, you can choose what to pay attention to, but your attention may also be drawn automatically by significant events.

Thus it would appear that attention is a series of mental processes enabled by specific areas within the brain. We engage our attention when we decide or are drawn to attend to a particular incoming stimulus; when we want to stop paying attention or turn our attention to something else, we disengage. Clinical research has shown that the thalamus is important for the so-called "engage function," and that the parietal lobe is involved in the disengage aspect. Meanwhile, the superior colliculus is responsible for the moving of attention. Finally, overall control of attention is thought to be controlled by an area of the brain called the anterior cingulate. Located in the frontal lobe near the center of the brain just in front of and above the lateral ventricles, the anterior cingulate is an important gyrus. Damage to any one of these areas can cause deficits in both voluntary and reflexive allocation of attention.

ADHD and autism

Brain damage is not the only source of attentional deficit. There are other conditions associated with attention deficits. Most notable are attention deficit

Parietal lobe
An area at the top of the brain important for spatial processing.

Superior colliculus
A thumbnail-sized cluster of neurons in the brain stem important for eye movements.

Gyrus
One of the convex folds on the surface of the brain, also called convolutions.

hyperactivity disorder (ADHD) and autism. People with autism seem to live in a private, self-absorbed world. They have marked social attentional deficits—they may fail to attend to their mother's face or voice or to others calling their name. ADHD has several characteristic patterns: one in which children simply cannot pay attention; another in which they show hyperactivity and impulsivity; and a third that combines the symptoms of the other two. Although ADHD and autism are distinctly different disorders, both have been shown to correlate with underdeveloped or underactive frontal lobes.

Memory and Mind

What happens after we selectively or reflexively attend to relevant information? We either relate it to previously acquired knowledge to recognize it, or we store it for later use. We remember millions of bits of information, some quite easily, others with difficulty. Why the big difference?

This question can be answered with reference to case studies of people with brain disorders who have deficits of memory. In the early 1950s the American neurosurgeon William Scoville developed a revolutionary surgical technique to cure epilepsy. Epilepsy is essentially caused by abnormal electrical activity in the brain. The condition can cause severe seizures, often resulting in loss of motor control and consciousness. Scoville's technique was called bilateral resection of the medial temporal lobe. This operation involved removing large parts of the middle portion of the temporal lobe on both sides of the brain.

Scoville's surgical operations were successful in alleviating the symptoms of epilepsy, but they had an unfortunate side effect. His patients came out of surgery without epilepsy but with severe and profound amnesia. Further, the severity of their

Curriculum Context

Students should understand the functions of the frontal lobes of the brain.

Amnesia

A partial or total inability to remember past events.

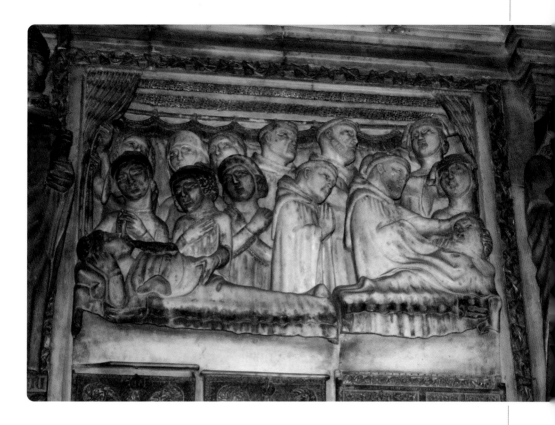

amnesia was directly proportional to the amount of the brain that had been removed.

The case of H. M.

The most famous case of this type was that of H. M., an epileptic who was operated on by Scoville and then became the subject of a long-term study. Twenty months after surgery it was obvious that H. M. had a memory deficit. When a specialist interviewed him, then left the room only to return a few minutes later, H. M. could not recall having met him before. He lacked the ability to form new memories of things that happened to him after the damage to his brain. H. M. could recall events that had happened to him before the operations (known as episodic memories), and he had retained some general knowledge (known as semantic memory). Nevertheless, he could not form new episodic or semantic memories.

Before the advent of modern drug treatment the only hope of a cure for epilepsy was prayer. This scene, where Saint Peter of Verona heals an epileptic, is in the Church of Sant' Eustorgia, in Milan, Italy.

Some researchers refer to the combination of episodic and semantic memories as explicit memories because they are usually memories that we know we know. There is also another sort of memory, those that we don't know we know, which are known as implicit memories. They include memories of procedural skills (such as driving a car), conditioning (such as salivating in expectation of food), and priming (for example, recognizing the word "dog" more quickly when it is preceded by the word "cat" than when it is preceded by the word "car"). One winter H. M. fell on ice and broke his hip. As he recovered, he became quite adept at folding and unfolding his portable walker (a procedural memory), but he couldn't remember sustaining the injury (which would have been an episodic memory). So H. M.'s implicit memory skills were relatively intact. This dissociation of explicit and implicit memories clearly demonstrates that memory is not a single, unitary system in the brain.

In addition to the disorders of the mind that are now linked with certainty to various forms of brain damage there are several other diseases that affect the mind.

Dementia caused by CJD

Creutzfeldt-Jacob disease (CJD) is an organic brain syndrome caused by a viruslike organism that results in dementia. CJD is one of a group of diseases called spongiform encephalopathies because it usually produces microscopic holes in brain tissue, giving it a spongelike appearance. It occurs in no more than about one person in half a million. However, the disease is fatal. Scientists are not sure exactly what causes it, or how it is contracted, and there is no known cure for the disease. It is known to be caused by a tiny protein particle called a prion that may be transmitted through ingestion of infected animal tissue.

Salivating

Secreting saliva, a watery liquid that aids chewing, swallowing, and digestion.

Dementia

The rapid, progressive deterioration of mental processes such as perception, attention, memory, motor processes, and language.

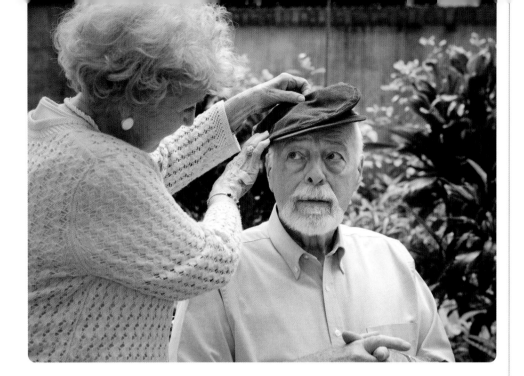

Dementia caused by Alzheimer's disease

A much more common disease that results in dementia is Alzheimer's disease. Like CJD, Alzheimer's is a degenerative disease of the brain from which there is no recovery. Slowly but surely, the disease damages many parts of the cerebral cortex and affects emotions, memory, language skills, reasoning, and motor processes. Again, scientists are not sure how the disease is caused. Alzheimer's may now be diagnosed through brain scans and cognitive tests.

Summing up

Most modern philosophers and neuroscientists agree that the mind is intrinsically linked to the brain. Clearly, mental processes such as attention, memory, and language are brain-based. We have seen how people with brain damage have mental deficits. Not all of these people can be described as having lost their minds but it can be said that they have lost portions of their mind. So it seems reasonable to conclude that the brain is the basis for our mental capabilities and is therefore the basis for what we call the human mind.

Alzheimer's begins with mild memory loss. Sufferers have trouble remembering recent events, activities, or the names of familiar people. These are all typical signs of aging and not in themselves necessarily anything to worry about, but in the case of Alzheimer's the symptoms progressively worsen.

Perception

The smell of toast and coffee. The feel of cool grass beneath our bare feet. Bird song. The blue of the sky. We recognize a whole range of colors and feelings, sounds and smells, because of our brain and its connections with our perceptual systems.

Sensation

The activity of special organs—eyes, ears, nose, tongue, and other sensors—that respond to things like heat, cold, and pressure.

Gland

An organ that secretes substances for use elsewhere in the body.

Curriculum Context

You may be asked to discuss how the use of new technologies provides information about the brain.

The world is filled with things that we can sense—that is, with forms of energy or structures that can be turned into sensation. Sensation alone would not be very meaningful without the brain, since it is nothing more than the transformation of physical stimuli into nerve impulses. It is the brain's interpretation of those impulses that allows us to perceive the colors, shapes, sounds, and feelings of the world in which we live.

James J. Gibson (1904–1979) argued that it is useful to consider sensation and perception together as making up our various perceptual systems. Those systems include not only the senses and the brain to which they are connected, but also muscles and glands.

The senses translate whatever is happening in the outside world into electrical nerve impulses that the brain can interpret. Only a small fraction of all available stimulation results in nerve impulses that the brain can interpret. Otherwise, we would be overwhelmed by our awareness of different sounds, sights, smells, tastes, and other sensations that surround us all the time.

Modern methods of research

The study of how the nervous system works is termed neuroscience. Research is based on findings from studies of human behavior, animals, neurological patients, and of neurology and anatomy.

Perhaps the most important fact is that neuroscientists now have sophisticated instruments that allow them to detect and map brain activity in ways not possible only a few decades ago. They can measure activity in single nerve cells and often identify specific areas of the brain that are involved when we respond to stimulation. Research reveals that there is an exceptionally close relationship between how we perceive and how we represent things in the brain.

Human vision

Our eyes are like an extension of our brains, pushed out toward the front of our heads along a stalk of nerve cells which keep our brain and eyes in constant contact. In fact, 40 percent of all the incoming nerve cells that connect our nervous system to the outside world come from the eyes.

Color vision

The retina of each eye contains about seven million cones but almost 20 times as many rods. Those light-sensitive cells are packed extremely tightly in an area about the size of a small postage stamp that is as thin as tissue paper. Rods are very sensitive to light. In fact, they are too sensitive to function well in normal light and are mainly for night vision. Cones need good light to function. They allow us to see details and colors.

Retina
The layer at the back of the eyeball containing cells that are sensitive to light.

Both rods and cones contain light-absorbing molecules that change as they absorb light. For example, rods contain the dim-light receptor rhodopsin, a chemical so sensitive that a single photon can break down a rhodopsin molecule. As the rhodopsin breaks down, it initiates a nerve signal. If the rod is to continue to respond to light, components of the rhodopsin need to recombine. It is because recombination needs to take place in the dark that rods do not function well in the daytime. The regeneration of rhodopsin dim-light receptors depends largely on vitamin A and certain proteins. Night blindness is common in areas where there is a shortage of foods containing vitamin A.

Photon
An elemental particle of light or other electromagnetic radiation.

Vitamin A
Retinol, a compound that is essential for growth and for low-light vision.

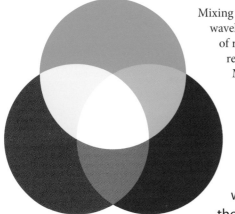

Mixing lights is an additive process. If we mix all wavelengths (or just the three primary colors of red, blue, and green), the effect is like recombining them to yield white light. Mixing pigments (like mixing paints) is different from mixing colored lights.

Theories of color vision

If you take all the colors of the rainbow and mix them, the result is white light. If you take only three of those colors—blue, green, and red—and combine them, the result is still white light. And if you combine pairs of those three colors, it is possible to generate all the colors that we can see.

The last of those facts is the basis for the trichromatic theory of color vision, proposed by Thomas Young (1773–1829) and expanded by Hermann Helmholtz (1821–1894). According to the Young–Helmholtz theory, it is possible to make all the colors we see simply by combining three different wavelengths—those of red, green, and blue—and the eye therefore needs only three kinds of color-sensitive cells. One kind would respond mainly to reds, one to greens, and the other to blues. Evidence that Young and Helmholtz might be right was first found in studies of people who are color-blind. In the end science determined that there are in fact three types of cones in the human retina: one responds mainly to longer wavelengths (reds), another to waves of intermediate length (greens), and a third to shorter waves (blues).

Color blindness

Since activity in three different types of cones allows us to see color, defects in one or more cone systems have predictable consequences. For example, people with no functioning cone systems see the world only in black, white, and shades of gray. They see poorly or not at all in daylight. People with only one functioning cone system see normally both by day and by night, but they cannot distinguish different colors because they see only different intensities of a single color. People with two functioning cone systems can see many colors, but they confuse certain colors that others distinguish easily. In many cases confusion is not total, and very bright colors can still be distinguished.

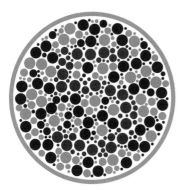 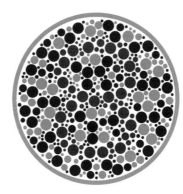

Two common tests for color blindness. If you are not color-blind, you will have little difficulty seeing the number 5 in the left-hand figure and the number 8 in the right-hand figure. People who are color blind need a stronger contrast in colors before they are able to read the figures.

The eyes and the brain

The eyes react to light waves, translating them into nerve signals that travel to the brain. It is the brain that interprets the information and perceives color, form, texture, and movement. The connection between eye and brain is the optic nerve. Signals from the right half of each eye go to the left side of the brain—called the left hemisphere; signals from the left half of each eye go to the opposite hemisphere—the right side of the brain. The main destination of visual signals is an area at the very back of the brain called the visual cortex, or the occipital lobe. The image in the retina is upside down and smaller than the actual object. The visual cortex turns it upright and interprets it in order to make it look like the original object.

To examine the role of the brain in visual perception investigators placed see-through goggles on the eyes of chimpanzees at birth. The goggles allowed light to enter; however, the animals were unable to see shapes

Curriculum Context

Many curricula expect students to be able to identify the neural pathways from the eyes to the brain.

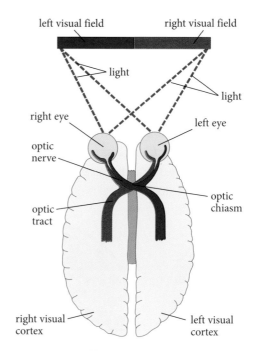

left visual field   right visual field

light

light

right eye

left eye

optic nerve

optic chiasm

optic tract

right visual cortex

left visual cortex

Images from the left visual field are transmitted to the right side of the brain, and images from the right visual field are transmitted to the left side of the brain. The visual cortex interprets and corrects them.

or patterns. Even after the goggles were removed, the chimpanzees required months before they could recognize objects or even guide their own movements in space. Most never achieved normal vision even after the goggles had been removed. It seems that early visual stimulation is essential for the development of normal visual perception.

Feature detectors

David Hubel and Thorsten Wiesel recorded the levels of brain activity in animals that had been deprived of visual stimulation. They found that many cells in the visual cortex seemed to have stopped functioning. In addition, there were far fewer connections between nerve cells in the visual cortex area of the brain. In one study the investigators reared cats with one eye sewn shut while the other one remained open. When they later removed the stitches so that both eyes could function, the visual cortex continued to respond only to the eye that had not been kept closed.

In some of their studies Hubel and Wiesel were able to record activity in single cells of the visual cortex. That allowed them to determine the effect on the retina of very specific stimulation, and they discovered that certain brain cells in the visual cortex are activated by very precise kinds of stimulation. For example, some respond only to lines of a certain width, and others to very specific angles or clear-cut movements. When those specialized cells, which are known as feature detectors, are not activated in the first weeks of life, many never function at all.

The Story of S. B.

The neuropsychologist Richard Gregory tells the story of S. B., a man who had been blind for the first 52 years of his life. During that time S. B. had adapted impressively. He rode confidently through his neighborhood on his bicycle with his hand on a friend's shoulder and he built things with tools in his own workshop. Then, at the age of 52 S. B. had corneal transplants. When the bandages were removed, he could see for the first time. But what he saw was a blurred and indistinct world. Although he soon learned to recognize familiar objects by sight, he developed little sense of perspective or depth and little understanding of speed or motion. So confused was he that he imagined he could easily lower himself to the ground from the window of his hospital room, not realizing it was more than 30 feet (9m) up! So uncertain was he of speed and distance that he became utterly terrified of crossing streets.

S. B. became increasingly depressed following his surgery, eventually spending long periods of time sitting alone at home in the dark. Some three years after the surgery S. B. died.

Recognizing faces and objects

As individuals we see only a very tiny fraction of this planet's six billion human faces, yet we would have no difficulty in identifying any one of them as an example of a human face. More than that, we instantly recognize hundreds of faces of people we know. Yet the differences between those faces are often so subtle that we cannot put them into words. Programmers find it hard to formulate the rules that would enable computers to detect important features and recognize familiar combinations. Our perceptual systems seem to have such feature detectors. They can identify several dozen important features for visual perception and even more sounds for auditory perception.

Gestalt principles

Recognizing complex forms such as faces or facial expressions seems to require a level of abstraction and decision making that is not very easily explained. According to the Gestalt psychologists, we perceive not individual features, but wholes. The foundation of Gestalt theory is that the whole is greater than the sum of its parts. Our brains are geared toward the best interpretation of the sensory information they receive.

Perceiving motion

When an object moves across our field of vision, it creates a series of images on the retina and we know it's moving. However, if you turn your head from left to right with your eyes open, you will have created a series of retinal images, but you won't see anything move. That's because your brain has compensated for your own movement. Similarly, if something moves by you and you move your head in perfect time with that object, there might not be a series of images created on your retina. But again, your brain compensates for your movement, and you know that the object has moved. Not everything that appears to move really does so. Motion pictures, for example, are sequences of still pictures that are presented so rapidly they give the appearance of movement. Other illusions are created by the brain's interpretation of perspective.

Hearing

Of all the senses, hearing is considered the most essential for spoken language. Many animal species depend far more on hearing than on sight for their communication, orientation, and survival. Dolphins cannot rely on their vision in the sometimes murky waters of their environment, but they do not really need to; neither do bats. Both these species make

Abstraction

The process of considering something independently of its attributes or associations.

Perspective

The suggestion of three dimensions in a two-dimensional medium.

Orientation

The determination of one's own position in relation to the surroundings.

The Blind Spot

There are no rods and cones in the area of the retina where the optic nerve joins the eyeball, resulting in a blind spot in our vision. You can demonstrate that by looking at the figure below. Hold the book 1 foot (30cm) or so in front of your face, close your right eye, and stare at the triangle on the right. Note how you can see the circle on the left even though you're staring at the triangle. Now move the book slowly back and forth. When the image hits your blind spot, the circle will disappear completely. Repeat the procedure described above, but this time pay attention to how the line that runs through the triangle and the circle looks solid and continuous even after the circle has disappeared. That is an important illustration of how we see not only with our eyes but also with our brains. Our brains expect the line to be continuous, so we see it that way.

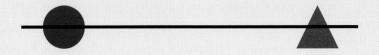

sounds that bounce off the objects around them and return to their hearing in the form of echoes. Nerve signals from their hearing to their brains enable them to build images of their worlds from the information they receive. Their finely controlled movements indicate a sophisticated spatial awareness.

The stimulus for sound

Sound is our perception of the effects of waves that are set off by vibrations. Sound waves involve the alternate compression and expansion of molecules—usually air molecules, but also molecules in liquids and solids. It is our perception of the waves that is the sound, not the waves themselves.

The creation and spread of sound waves are similar to what would happen if you threw a pebble into a calm pond. You would see how ripples start where the pebble enters the water and how they fan out in ever-widening circles. The ripples are created at a fixed rate—a number of them pass a certain point each second. That is their frequency. Frequency does not change as the waves fan out. Frequency of sound waves is measured in Hertz (Hz) units. The human ear is sensitive to frequencies between 16 and 20,000 Hz, provided they are loud enough. The lower the frequency, the lower the pitch (tone) we perceive.

To consider the pond again, the waves closest to where the pebble hits will have higher peaks than more distant waves. Amplitude is the height of a wave. Amplitude decreases as distance increases until the waves stop altogether. In the case of sound, amplitude, or loudness, is measured in decibels. Zero decibels is the approximate lower threshold of our hearing. Very high intensities can be dangerous. More than eight hours of exposure to sounds at 100 decibels can permanently damage hearing.

If you threw two pebbles into the pond, waves would fan out from each pebble, crashing into each other to create a network of little wavelets. Those wavelets could no longer be described in terms of frequency and amplitude alone because they would be too complex. Complexity is the third characteristic of sound waves. The sound waves that surround us are not usually pure sounds from one source; more often they are combinations of sounds.

Structure of the ear

The visible part of the human ear is the pinna, a piece of flesh that spirals like a question mark into either side of your head. The pinna, together with the short, wax-filled auditory canal, which conducts vibrations from the pinna to the eardrum, is part of the outer ear.

The middle ear is a small, air-filled cavity containing three tiny bones (ossicles): the hammer (malleus) is connected directly to the eardrum at one end and to the anvil (incus) at the other. The anvil, in turn,

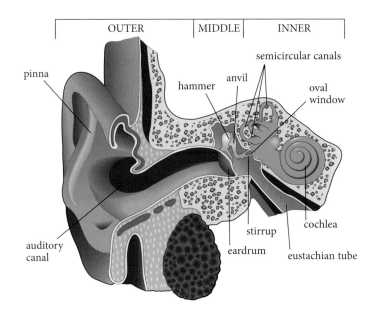

OUTER | MIDDLE | INNER

pinna

semicircular canals

hammer

anvil

oval window

auditory canal

stirrup

cochlea

eardrum

eustachian tube

The three main parts of the ear are the outer, middle, and inner sections. Within this overall structure the ear is a complex collection of tubes, canals, containers, fluids, membranes, bones, cartilage, and nerves.

connects with the stirrup (stapes). The stirrup fits over a small membrane (oval window) that leads to the inner ear. There is also a passage, the eustachian (auditory) tube, that leads from the middle ear to the throat.

The inner ear contains the cochlea, a fluid-filled structure shaped like a snail's shell. Inside the cochlea is the basilar membrane, along which are the sound-receptive hair cells that make up the organ of Corti.

How the ear works

Sound waves are funneled by the pinna through the auditory canal, causing the eardrum in the middle ear to vibrate. Although the vibrations are very slight, they set up corresponding vibrations in the three little bones of the middle ear, which are then transmitted to the inner ear via the oval window. Movement of the oval window causes movement in the fluids of the inner ear, setting up wavelike motions of the basilar membrane. They cause the hair cells of the organ of Corti to move. As those cells bend and twist, they activate nerve cells at their base. Impulses in those nerve cells are then transmitted to both hemispheres of the brain via the auditory nerve.

Curriculum Context

Students should understand the function of each part of the ear.

Locating sounds

Many sound waves reach our two ears at slightly different times. If the sound comes directly from one side, it will reach the farther ear about 0.8 milliseconds later than it reaches the nearer ear. In addition, the nearer ear receives the vibrations directly; the vibrations are less intense when they reach the farther ear because they have been diverted around the head. If the sound comes directly from above, in front, or behind, it reaches both ears at about the same time and with the same intensity. But the shape of the pinna changes the waves in different ways depending on the direction from which they come. We use these cues—time difference, intensity difference, and distortions resulting from the angle at which the vibrations strike the ear—to judge the direction of a sound.

Our ability to perceive and process different pitches not only helps us to survive and communicate; it also allows us to enjoy and make sense of complex musical sounds.

Perceiving pitch

In daily life we need to be able to detect, learn, and recognize sounds. For that we need to be able to perceive pitch. One theory, the frequency theory, suggests that sound waves give rise to brain activity that corresponds directly to the frequency of the wave.

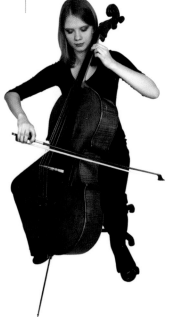

In other words, a wave at 500 cycles per second (500 Hz) would give rise to 500 nerve impulses per second. There is evidence that this does happen, but only for the lower frequencies, because a nerve cannot ordinarily fire more than about 1,000 times per second. A second explanation, called place theory, suggests that high and low frequencies affect different parts of the cochlea. If the base of the cochlea is most active, we hear higher frequencies; if the upper end is most active, we perceive lower frequencies.

Hearing and language

Spoken language is hearing's most important contribution to our lives. Its evolutionary significance can hardly be overstated; neither can its contribution to our thinking and to our ability to solve problems and to adapt. In oral (spoken) language we use sounds for which we have widespread agreement concerning their referents (meanings). But language can also consist of visual rather than auditory symbols—now, for example, you are reading the words written on the page. Language can also consist mainly of gestures.

Spoken language depends on our hearing. Information from each ear is transmitted via the auditory nerve to either side of the brain. Our brains hear and process sounds. How the brain associates sounds with meanings is still a matter of speculation, but scientists do know where in the brain that activity takes place.

Research on brain activity

In 1861 Paul Broca (1824–1880) performed an autopsy on a patient with a severe speech disorder. He found

Autopsy
An examination of a dead body to discover the cause of death or the extent of disease.

The Basic Orienting System

There is a complex structure in our inner ears that has nothing to do with hearing. It lies in the part of the ear named the labyrinth, which includes the snail-shell-shaped cochlea and three other tubes called semicircular canals. The tubes are set at right angles to each other and are filled with fluid. They are the main sense organs of our basic orienting system that detects bodily movement and position.

When we move, lie down, spin, or stand on our heads, the fluid in our semicircular canals moves in expected ways. Hair cells inside the canals translate the effects of those movements into nerve impulses that our brains interpret to determine that we are doing those things— moving, lying down, spinning, or standing on our heads. Our basic orienting system relies not only on our inner-ear receptors, but also on sensations we get from receptors in our muscles, tendons, and joints (our kinesthetic senses). The kinesthetic senses allow our brains to know that our arms and legs are bent this way or that, or that we are moving forward or backward. In addition, our other perceptual systems are brought into play. For example, we know when we are moving because sensors in our muscles and joints or movements of the fluid in our semicircular canals tell us so. Our visual system also tells us that we are moving. Some aspects of movement are coded by specific cells in the visual cortex, and these cells respond to particular aspects such as speed or direction.

damage to a small area on the left side of the frontal lobe of his brain. Broca correctly concluded that the injury explained the man's inability to produce the ordinary sounds of language. That area of the brain is now known as Broca's area. A short time later Carl Wernicke (1848–1905) identified another area on the left-hand side of the brain—now known as Wernicke's area—that is closely related to the production of speech. Very close to Wernicke's area is a third structure, the angular gyrus, which is also involved in language. It is generally agreed that in most people the left hemisphere is more dedicated to language than the right one.

Event-related potentials

Electroencephalograms (EEGs), positron emission tomography (PET scans), and functional magnetic resonance imaging (fMRI) give information about brain activity either in the entire brain or in regions of the brain. EEGs give general recordings of brain activity; PET scans show the level of activity in different regions of the brain; and fMRI provides a picture of nerve activity in various structures of the brain.

When EEG recordings are taken while a person is exposed to a special stimulus, it is possible to detect electrical activity that relates directly to that stimulus. That activity is called an event-related potential (ERP). ERPs are now among the most often studied variables in brain research. Some studies show that responses to spoken words as well as responses associated with producing words are stronger in the left hemisphere than in the right. Nevertheless, ERPs in response to stimulation of hearing tend to occur in both hemispheres. And when signals are fed into only one ear, the ERP is usually stronger in the opposite hemisphere. Those findings support both the conclusion that the left hemisphere is very involved in language and the general principle of contralaterality.

Variable

Something whose value is subject to change.

Contralaterality

The principle that each brain hemisphere tends to control functioning in the opposite side of the body.

Although we know that Broca's area is involved in producing speech and Wernicke's area in understanding speech, ERP research shows that many other areas of the brain participate in those processes. The nerve architecture that underlies language is complex and not yet very clear. For example, ERPs produced by auditory signals occur earliest in the brain stem and then in several other brain structures before they occur in the auditory cortex. In addition, ERPs arise not only in response to external stimuli; they also happen in response to thoughts and emotions that are independent of external stimulation. ERP research may eventually tell us much more than we now know about the specific areas of the brain involved in different perceptual, mental, and physical processes.

Curriculum Context

Students should be able to identify the areas of the brain involved in perception of sound and language.

The body senses

We know much more about seeing and hearing than we do about our other senses. Yet those other senses are very important to our functioning. Take, for example, the body senses, sometimes known as the somesthetic senses. Among other things, they are essential for moving around, for staying upright or knowing about body position, and for avoiding things that are painful and that might damage or kill us.

Three Is Soft and Yellow: Synesthesia

Normally our senses, our perceptual antennas, are tuned to different features of our world. They give us separate but related images of the same scene. But some people have a rare condition termed synesthesia in which stimulation of one perceptual system leads to their experiencing imagery in another.

The most common forms of synesthesia involve visual images. The images are usually highly consistent and predictable. Some people see colors or other visual images when they feel certain moods or when they are in pain. Still others feel tactile (touch) sensations when they hear music. We have no widely accepted explanation for synesthesia in spite of a spurt of recent research. It is possible that some artists experience especially rich mental imagery because they have the condition.

Touch: the haptic system

The word *haptic* comes from the Greek meaning "to be able to lay hold of"—hence its use for the sense of touch. The haptic perceptual system is also called the skin senses. They consist of various receptors that give us information about bodily contact. Some receptors are sensitive to pressure; others react to warmth and cold; still others provide sensations of pain. The senses rely on more than one million nerve cells that have endings in or near the epidermis.

Epidermis

The outer layer of the skin.

Temperature

Two kinds of receptors allow us to sense changes in temperature, one kind sensitive to heat and the other to cold. Cold receptors increase their rate of firing when the temperature is dropping; heat receptors increase theirs when temperature climbs. Information from cold and heat receptors is essential to our brains if they are to maintain our body temperatures within a normal range. The brain readjusts our temperature by sending out signals that lead to blood-vessel dilation and increased perspiration when we're too warm or blood-vessel constriction when we're too cold.

Pain

One of the functions of pain is to keep us from doing things that are harmful—like walking on broken glass or leaning on a hot stove. Pain results from the stimulation of nerve endings (pain receptors) by pressure, heat, or sometimes chemicals. There are also pain receptors in the internal organs. When they are stimulated, we feel visceral pain. This is often felt in parts of the body that are far removed from the true source of the pain. For example, people suffering from heart pain may have the sensation of pain in their arm, their neck, or perhaps even in their hand.

Two distinct types of nerve pathways transmit pain sensations to the brain. The first, transmitted by the rapid nerve pathways, is the instant, sharp pain you feel when you first burn your hand. The pain message reaches your brain very rapidly and is sharp and insistent because its function is to make you pull away from the cause of it in time to prevent serious damage. The response is swift and automatic. The second type of pain sensation, which is transmitted by the slower pathways, is the dull ache that continues after you have pulled away.

Curriculum Context

Some curricula expect students to be able to explain perception in the human haptic system.

One explanation of how the body processes pain is the gate-control theory proposed by Ronald Melzack and P. D. Wall. According to them, we feel pain when the nerve cells that connect pain receptors to the brain are active. Those nerve cells, called C-fibers, have to pass through a series of "gates" to reach the brain. However, those gates are not always fully open and are sometimes completely shut. That is because there is a second kind of nerve cell, called an A-fiber, that can close some of the gates, preventing the passage of pain signals. C-fibers, which carry pain signals, transmit at a faster rate than A-fibers, which hinder pain sensations. So we quickly sense sharp pain when we

Phantom Limb Pain

Psychologist Krista Wilkins and her associates studied 60 children and adolescents who lacked a limb. Nearly half of them had been born with a missing limb; the others had undergone surgical amputation. Only a small fraction of those born with a missing limb experienced phantom sensations. But even after their surgery had healed, almost 70 percent of the amputees had phantom pain. Some of them had stump pain, where the site of the surgery itself hurt. But many also had phantom limb pain in which the pain seemed to be located in the absent limb. For more than a third of those amputees phantom limb pain mirrored the pain they had felt in the limb before surgery. Phantom limb pain is real pain. Patterns of brain activity are much the same in people experiencing pain in a missing limb as they are in people experiencing pain in a real limb. That seems to be evidence that phantom limb sensations are produced in the brain by the same processes that underlie other sensations of pain, but without the external stimuli.

hurt ourselves. The "neural gate" involves a region of the midbrain, where neurons inhibit the cells that would normally communicate pain. When the neurons are active, the neural gate is closed; and when the neurons are not active, the neural gate is open.

The chemical senses

Taste (gustation) and smell (olfaction) are essential for survival. They prevent us poisoning ourselves and entice us to eat. The organ that makes it possible for us to smell is the olfactory epithelium, which is located toward the top of our nasal (nose) passages. It is a small membrane covered by a mat of tiny hairlike structures called cilia. The hairs respond to molecules dissolved in the mucus (thick, slimy fluid) lining the nasal passages, transmitting impulses directly to the olfactory bulb, a small protrusion at the front underside of the brain above the olfactory epithelium.

We cannot easily describe what something smells like other than by comparing it to other objects with strong and familiar odors. Research indicates that we often have powerful recollections of odors and strong associations with them. And it seems that we can distinguish more than 10,000 different smells. The part

Curriculum Context

Students should be able to explain how the olfactory sensory system operates.

A side view of the nose showing the olfactory epithelium and the olfactory bulb. The ability to detect odors depends on cilia, hairlike extensions of the cells that make up the olfactory epithelium. The olfactory bulb, the brain organ involved in olfaction, is immediately above the olfactory epithelium.

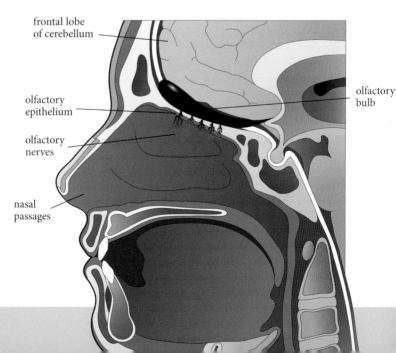

frontal lobe of cerebellum

olfactory epithelium

olfactory nerves

nasal passages

olfactory bulb

of our brain devoted to smell is very small in comparison with the total size of our brain; in contrast, about one-third of a dog's cortex is involved in smell. Some scientists estimate that a dog's sense of smell is one million times more powerful than that of a person.

Pheromones

A male moth flitting around on a dark night might suddenly become aware of a female moth several miles away. A dog's nose tells him the exact location of a neighboring bitch in heat. Almost all receptive female animals give off airborne molecules called pheromones, which are highly attractive to the male of the species.

Scientists have tried to find human sexual pheromones. We know there are human secretions that are pheromonelike—on male armpit hair and in urine. Some studies have shown that females are more sensitive to those substances than are males, especially when they are releasing eggs (ovulating). Some research also indicates that exposure to pheromones may positively affect women's moods. But no clear link has yet been found between human pheromonelike substances and sexual behavior.

Gustation

Taste depends on chemicals being dissolved in fluids that surround taste-sensitive cells. Those cells are on the tongue in clusters of about 40 or 50, in protrusions known as taste buds. The taste buds are dotted with tiny openings through which dissolved chemicals reach the taste cells. Taste cells have a life cycle of only about 4 to 10 days, after which they die and are regenerated.

Our language for taste is no more exact than that for smell. We might simply say that something is sweet, sour, salty, bitter, or some combination of those terms. It seems that different parts of the tongue are more sensitive to each of those tastes. Smell is sometimes more important than the reaction of our taste buds in the tasting of food. If you were to pinch your nose tightly while taking alternate bites of an apple and an onion, you would be unlikely to detect any difference in taste between the two.

Emotion and Motivation

Emotions play a vital role in everyday life and in mental health. Although many advances have been made in our understanding of emotions, we are still just beginning to unravel the complex relationship between emotions and the body.

Physiological

Concerning the way living organisms and their body parts work.

Any emotion has three components: Physiological changes, such as acceleration of heart rate and activation of specific regions in the brain; behavioral responses, such as a tendency to escape from or prolong contact with whatever is causing the emotion; and a subjective experience, such as feeling angry, happy, or sad about the person or thing causing the emotion. Emotions are therefore a specific and automatic set of consciously experienced responses in reaction to a real or imagined stimulus.

Evolution

The process by which different organisms are thought to have developed, over time, from earlier forms.

The functions of emotions

In 1872 Charles Darwin argued that emotions are a beneficial product of evolution. He believed that species retain their emotional capabilities during evolution because they play an important role in communication, which improves chances of survival. According to Darwin, each emotion that was important for survival developed a very specific type of expression. In humans two aspects of expression are most important: facial expressions and behavior.

The expression of emotions helps in our social life by allowing us to communicate quickly. Experimental studies have shown that people can accurately recognize other people's emotional states merely by glancing at their faces. However, failures to recognize emotions accurately can have severe consequences. Anyone who is unable to tell these different emotions apart is at a great social disadvantage.

Today psychologists assume that emotions have an important adaptive function, enabling people to adjust to new circumstances. One of the ways this comes about is through providing motivational impetus. Emotions allow individuals of any species to make an instant, possibly life-saving, response to events. Emotions provide clear goals to pursue. In addition to telling you what to do to survive in a dangerous situation, emotions also mobilize the energy you need to carry out these behaviors. The experience of emotion includes changes in the activity of the autonomic nervous system. A feeling of fear, for example, causes the autonomic system to increase the heart rate and blood pressure. That supplies the muscles of the voluntary system with the oxygen and glucose they need to move you speedily away from danger.

Emotions also guide your attention toward important stimuli and provide a stream of information about whether or not you have attained your action goals, such as escape. They provide fast, clear communication about current stimuli and goals and energy for behavior, as well as telling the person what to do. Emotions therefore help ensure survival.

Are basic emotions innate?

In this functional view of emotions there is a set of basic emotions shared by all humans that are important for the survival of the species. There is strong evidence that basic emotions are innate (inborn), rather than learned. For example, people who are born blind and have never seen faces still display the typical facial expressions of the basic emotions.

In 1983 Paul Ekman, Robert Levenson, and Wallace Friesen asked people to adjust their face muscles to show a particular basic emotion. At the same time, they assessed several physiological factors relating to the

Autonomic nervous system

The communication network by which the brain controls all parts of the body except for contraction of skeletal muscles

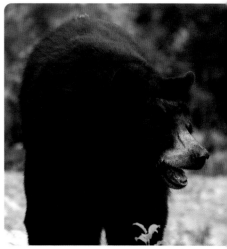

Meeting this large black bear would probably elicit the startle response followed by a complex mixture of physiological, behavioral, and subjective reactions.

activation of the autonomous nervous system. They found clear evidence that the expression of different emotions is accompanied by different adjustments of the nervous system. This finding suggested that there is a link between the facial expression of a basic emotion and how the body prepares itself for action. However, few studies of the autonomic nervous system have confirmed such active links between facial expression and autonomic responses.

Basic Emotions

In 1971 Paul Ekman and Wallace Friesen tested whether facial expressions of emotion are shared universally among all humans. They showed photographs of Americans portraying different emotions to people from a variety of cultures, including New Guinea tribes, and asked them to identify the emotion. The results suggested that expressions of six "basic" emotions—happiness, fear, anger, sadness, disgust, and surprise—are indeed shared irrespective of culture.

In 1980 Robert Plutchik proposed a new view of emotions. His model included eight primary innate emotions: joy, acceptance, fear, surprise, sadness, disgust, anger, and anticipation. According to Plutchik, all these primary emotions have an important role in survival because they are linked to distinct behavioral programs, such as "destruction" in the case of anger or "approach" in the case of joy. Plutchik also suggested that complex emotions such as guilt and love are derived from combinations of primary emotions.

One criticism of the idea of basic emotion has come from the observation that people from different cultures do not always express the same basic emotions in quite the same way.

Other evidence has led to further criticism of the idea that humans share a fixed set of basic emotions. In 1995 James Russell reported studies in which he and

Curriculum Context

Students can usefully compare and contrast Plutchik's and Russell's theories of primary emotions.

Private and Public Behavior

To demonstrate that people react differently in public and private settings, Ekman and Friesen showed different stressful film clips to Americans and Japanese, and recorded their facial expressions. The participants watched the film clips either alone or in the presence of an experimenter of the same ethnic group. When they were alone, the participants showed similar expressions; but when the experimenter later interviewed them while they were watching a replay of the film clips, the Japanese participants tended to mask their responses more than the Americans, providing evidence of cultural differences in display rules.

his colleagues presented pictures of mimed facial expressions to participants in the study. He found that people only described these facial expressions in two basic ways: pleasure–displeasure and calmness–arousal.

The emotional circumplex

Russell's two-dimensional theory was not new, however. More than 100 years ago Wilhelm Wundt suggested that all emotional experiences can be classified using the dimensions of pleasure and arousal. This model, called the emotional circumplex, has become the main alternative to explaining emotion in terms of a set of basic emotions.

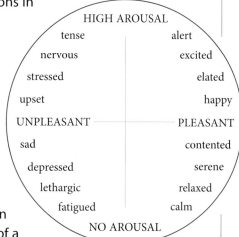

In 1988 Peter Lang and his colleagues published a large set of emotion-provoking pictures that were rated on the dimensions of pleasure (pleasant or unpleasant) and arousal (calming or emotion-arousing). Lang used the pictures in a study in which he noted both the viewers' subjective ratings of arousal and pleasantness and objective measurements of their autonomic nervous system activity. When Lang compared participants' own ratings of their emotional reactions to the

Russell's circumplex model of emotions. According to Russell, emotions can be represented as a combination of degrees along two dimensions—arousal and unpleasantness—rather than by basic emotions. For example, a feeling of elation combines high degrees of arousal and pleasantness.

physiological measurements, he found a high rate of agreement between them.

Causes of emotions

According to common wisdom, all your responses to a situation occur because you experience an emotion. However, William James turned this idea on its head. For example, according to James' theory of emotions, your conscious fear is the result of your physical reactions to the threat, not the other way around. Your heart pounds, you stop still, and you feel fear. In short, James proposed that feeling an emotion only becomes possible through changes in the body.

The "facial feedback hypothesis" has been formulated by researchers influenced by James' idea. Jim Laird has conducted several studies of this hypothesis. The studies show that if people adjust their facial muscles to match how they would be during the expression of an emotion, they actually feel that emotion.

Walter Cannon conducted studies of the autonomic nervous system during the 1920s. According to his research, visceral changes in response to emotional stimuli occur far more slowly than the associated feeling. He found no evidence for specific patterns of visceral changes linked to particular emotions. Cannon concluded that James' order of events had to be wrong and suggested that a stressful stimulus first creates an emergency reaction in the brain—a state of general arousal that prepares the body for a "fight or flight" response to the negative stimulus whatever its nature. At the same time, a conscious emotion is generated.

At the beginning of the 1960s Stanley Schachter developed a kind of compromise between the views of James and Cannon. According to Schachter, any significant event in the environment can create a state of general, unspecific arousal in the autonomic

Visceral

Relating to the viscera—the organs within the chest and abdomen.

Curriculum Context

Students should be aware of the differences between James' and Cannon's ideas of what triggers emotional reactions.

nervous system. According to Schachter, when people experience arousal and their heart pounds, for example, they ask themselves why that is happening; the specific emotion they then feel and express depends on the explanation they find.

Choosing our Emotions

In the early 1960s Stanley Schachter and Jerome Sugar conducted experiments to prove that bodily arousal is only linked with emotions when people believe the arousal is caused by external situations.

In one experiment he divided the participants into two groups, giving one group an injection of the drug epinephrine (which speeds up the heart and breathing) and the other group a placebo (an inactive substance). Only some of the epinephrine-injected individuals were informed of the effects of the drug. The participants were then exposed to a situation likely to elicit an emotional response: They were insulted or amused. From their reported responses and behavioral expressions it was clear that the epinephrine-injected individuals who were unaware of the effects of the drug they had been given had experienced more intense emotion and fear than either the placebo group or the informed epinephrine-injected group. They attributed their heightened state to the qualities of the stimuli to which they were exposed; they felt anger at the insults, for example, while the other groups felt only irritation. The group of epinephrine-injected individuals who understood the drug's effects attributed their jittery feelings to the drug, and their responses to the stimuli were similar to those of the placebo group. Schachter's experiment suggests that we experience arousal, we interpret it, and then the emotion occurs, in that order.

Cognition and emotion

Some researchers focused on the question "What makes a stimulus provoke an emotion?" For them cognition became more important than body processes. Around 1960 Magda Arnold introduced the concept of appraisal. According to this cognitive approach, the way people appraise a situation determines the emotion they ultimately experience.

There are often big differences in how people feel and respond to the same stimuli. According to appraisal theory, that is because people differ in their

Cognition
The processing of information by the brain.

Appraisal
The subjective assessment of the potential harm or benefit of a situation.

Curriculum Context

Appraisal theory is one of the cognitive theories of emotion that many curricula expect students to be aware of.

evaluation of the situation. People feel an emotion when they achieve conscious access to the appraisal's outcome. Arnold also introduced the idea of action tendencies—behavioral impulses, like fleeing or fighting, that can become real actions. They can also determine emotional responses to a stimulus or an event.

Bernard Weiner proposed that emotions are the result of mental strategies for processing information. This approach focused on complex emotions such as guilt and pride, which are concerned with evaluations of the self and others. According to Weiner, an emotional reaction to an event depends on the causes a person finds for the event rather than on the event itself.

Society and emotions

In the 1980s a new perspective called social constructivism moved the foundations of emotions further away from biology and firmly in the direction of cognition (where activity in the brain's cortex is held responsible for the generation of emotions). According to this theory, emotions are the product of the rules and scripts that a society creates to predict reactions to events. The rules and scripts determine the way that people interpret events, and they signal which kinds of emotional reaction are appropriate and which are not.

Emotions and the unconscious

In 1980 Robert Zajonc argued that emotional reactions to stimuli are evoked faster and more spontaneously than cognitive theories could explain. Further, we can often say how we feel about a situation before we know what we think about it. Cognition and emotion must therefore be distinct and independent processes.

Zajonc reported the results of several experiments on the effect of prior exposure to a stimulus on people's reaction to it. For example, Zajonc presented his participants with a series of unfamiliar Chinese ideograms and then assessed how much they liked or disliked them. He found that the more frequently one particular ideogram was presented, the more it was liked by the participants.

The "mere exposure" effect occurred even when stimuli were presented for a few milliseconds, when it was impossible for the participants to consciously recognize the stimuli. The ideograms were later presented for longer periods, and participants judged how much they liked them. The results showed that previously seen ideograms are perceived as more likable. People therefore can form basic emotional reactions, such as an attitude toward an object without having any conscious awareness of it.

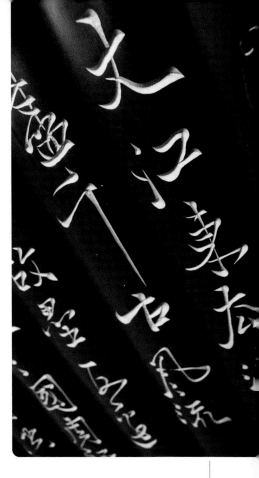

In later studies participants were momentarily shown a stimulus with emotional impact: a drawing of either a frowning or smiling face. The initial stimuli were shown so quickly that it was impossible to recognize them consciously. Immediately after this exposure, participants were briefly shown an unfamiliar stimulus, such as a Chinese ideogram. Finally, the second stimuli were presented again, and participants were asked how much they liked them. The results showed that people liked the ideograms more if they appeared after a smiling face than after a frowning face.

Robert Zajonc used Chinese ideograms like these in experiments to test whether people would develop a preference for neutral, unfamiliar stimuli through brief exposure to them.

Emotions and the brain
Since the 1930s researchers have tried to discover the areas of the brain responsible for different functions, including the mechanisms of escape and aggression. In general, each area of the brain is involved in more than

one function, with various regions and structures working together to carry out functions.

An unknown number of different brain areas play a part in producing emotions. Different species show the same emotional behaviors suggesting that regions that coordinate emotions developed early in the brain's evolution. So the cortex, which evolved relatively late, is not the place to look for the seat of the emotions. We need to look in the older parts of the brain.

The Case of Fear

Fear was one of the first emotions to be investigated systematically by scientists, and it is probably the best understood emotion. Fear reactions allow an animal to protect itself.

In such fear reactions one region of the brain—the amygdala—seems to be especially important. When an animal perceives itself to be in a dangerous situation, the perception of danger passes from the sensory thalamus directly to the amygdala via the "low road." The amygdala activates a sequence of hormone releases, first from the hypothalamus. This releases hormones that trigger the pituitary gland to produce a further hormone that causes the adrenal glands to release steroid hormones. They activate neurons in the hippocampus, amygdala, and other areas. This complex circuit of hormone releases continues until the dangerous stimulus disappears. At the same time, information about the stimulus travels via the "high road" to the sensory cortex, which makes an evaluation of the stimulus and sends it to the amygdala. If the cortex concludes that there is cause for fear, the amygdala is instructed to continue initiating the hormonal sequence, triggering escape or confrontation. If the cortex judges the threat to be past or false, it instructs the amygdala to stop the hormonal sequence, and the animal relaxes.

The autonomic nervous system is controlled by such older parts of the brain. It is divided into a sympathetic branch responsible for activation of systems of the body, such as the heart and blood circulation and breathing, and a parasympathetic branch responsible for deactivation of the systems to resting levels of activity. Sympathetic and parasympathetic discharges (electrical signals passed on by nerve cells) prompt responses in several organs. Neurotransmitters, or chemical messengers, called adrenaline and noradrenaline are released into the bloodstream when the sympathetic nervous system is aroused. The discharge galvanizes people into responding physically to the challenges they face. Release of acetylcholine by parasympathetic fibers occurs when the body disengages from the stressful situation and is freed to relax. The autonomic nervous system, therefore, plays a vital role in instigating and carrying out behaviors and thus expressing emotions in a physical way.

The part of the brain that plays an important part in control of the autonomic nervous system is called the medulla, which is in the brain stem, at the base of the brain. Electrical stimulation of one part of the medulla, the rostral portion, evokes sympathetic arousal all over the body, while stimulation of another part, the vagal nucleus, evokes parasympathetic discharge. The medulla is influenced by parts of the higher brain stem that project down to it, namely, the hypothalamus and the amygdala, and regions of the cortex. All of these areas play a role in emotions.

Curriculum Context

Students should be able to understand how the sympathetic and parasympathetic nervous systems work on heart rate in an emotional situation.

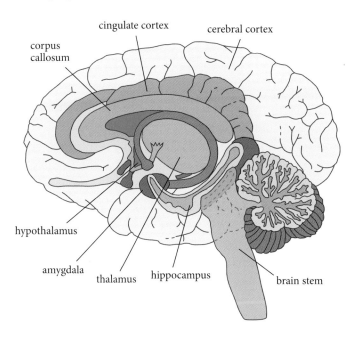

corpus callosum

cingulate cortex

cerebral cortex

hypothalamus

amygdala

thalamus

hippocampus

brain stem

Many areas of the brain are involved in emotional perception and response. These brain areas are not exclusively concerned with emotions, but also have important roles in relation to other functions.

Researchers have used animals to further knowledge of the deeper brain regions. In one type of study researchers electrically stimulate certain areas of the brain until a behavior is evoked. Another method, called a lesion study, involves systematically destroying parts of the brain with lesions until an emotional behavior disappears. Investigation of people with brain damage is another long-used method of studying the human brain. Researchers test which abilities are limited or absent after brain injuries.

In addition to these methods the human brain is investigated using imaging technologies such as fMRI, a form of magnetic resonance imaging in which the brain's activity can be viewed as it is taking place. Also used is positron emission tomography (PET), in which very short-lived radioisotopes are introduced into the brain, and a computer is used to analyze the gamma rays emitted by them. Such techniques make visible the activated regions of the brain.

Models of the emotional brain

Researchers have also tried to find the pathway of emotions within the brain. William James' theory connected two parts of the cerebral cortex: the sensory cortex and the motor cortex. According to James, an emotional stimulus enters the sensory cortex, where it is perceived. From the sensory cortex the information about the stimulus passes to the motor cortex. This produces a bodily response. The bodily response feeds back to the cortex, which recognizes that the body is moving. The perception of the bodily response is what we experience as emotional feeling. In short, James reasoned that the critical brain pathways are connections between cortical areas, and the brain does not possess a specific emotion system.

Walter Cannon and Philip Bard criticized both of these assumptions. Around 1920 Philip Bard conducted a series of lesion studies with cats to research anger and rage. Cats still showed clear signs of emotional arousal after their cortex had been removed. Exposed to threatening or provocative stimuli, they were still able to react with aggression accompanied by high autonomic arousal—the emergency reaction. Their reactions were more intense than those of cats with complete brains, probably because the reactions had not been tempered by the cortex.

Bard found that the hypothalamus was the critical brain structure for the expression of anger. This structure plays a very important role in the control of autonomic nervous system responses involved in the "fight or flight" response. Removal of the hypothalamus in cats results in an inability to show a coordinated anger response. Electrical stimulation of the hypothalamus results in rage reactions.

The pathway Cannon and Bard proposed runs as follows. On its way to the relevant cortical areas, sensory information passes the thalamus with its specialized regions for sensory inputs. From there information proceeds to the hypothalamus and the cerebral cortex at the same time. As soon as the hypothalamus receives signals, it activates body responses that may be seen in the expression of emotions. Simultaneously, the hypothalamus sends signals to the cerebral cortex, indicating that emotional arousal has been provoked. That information is integrated with sensory information about the stimulus coming directly from the thalamus to the cortex, with the result that an emotional feeling is experienced.

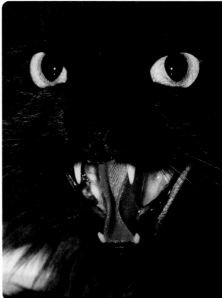

A cat showing aggression when faced with a threatening situation. In the 1920s researchers into anger and rage discovered that even when cats had their whole cortex removed, they still showed these emotions. This suggests that important pathways of emotion reside in the deeper brain structures rather than in the cortex.

The circuit theory
In 1937 James Papez drew a more detailed map of the emotional pathways in the brain. Emotional feeling is

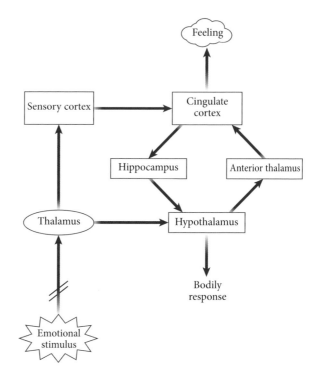

The Papez circuit theory. Papez' theory was far more specific than Cannon and Bard's about how the hypothalamus communicates with the brain and which areas of the brain are involved.

created in the cingulate cortex, an older structure in the middle axis of the brain, which integrates inputs from the sensory cortex and the hypothalamus.

According to Papez, there are two pathways to the cortex. The first is the "stream of thinking" from the thalamus via the sensory cortex to the cingulate cortex. The second is the "stream of feeling" from the thalamus to the cingulate cortex via the hypothalamus. The hypothalamus sends input to the anterior thalamus (the organ's frontal area). From there signals reach the cingulate cortex. At the same time, the cingulate cortex receives information about the emotional stimulus from the sensory cortex and integrates this information with the input from the anterior thalamus.

Papez also considered a possible pathway through which the brain can control emotional responses: from the cingulate cortex via the hippocampus back to the hypothalamus. This pathway opened the door to explaining how internal "thoughts" can create emotions. Areas of the cerebral cortex involved in

Curriculum Context

Many curricula expect students to understand the emotional pathways of communication in the brain.

perception and memory can also activate the cingulate cortex, which activates the hypothalamus via the hippocampus.

The limbic system model

From the work of Heinrich Klüver and Paul Bucy it was known that the tiny structure called the amygdala seemed to have a role in producing aggressive response to stimuli. For example, destruction of the amygdala in wild monkeys made them placid, while electrical stimulation of the amygdala in a cat would produce either an attack or a fear response. These findings influenced Paul MacLean when he formulated his limbic system theory of emotions in 1949.

MacLean emphasized the role of the hypothalamus in the physical manifestations of emotions, as well as the importance of the cerebral cortex in emotional feelings. His goal was to discover how those regions of the brain communicate with one another. The neocortex is not connected with the hypothalamus, but it is connected with part of the older medial cortex called the rhinencephalon, or smell brain. MacLean believed that the part of the brain concerned with smell was also the seat of emotions. Because electrical stimulation of this region resulted in autonomic nervous system responses, Maclean introduced the term "visceral brain" for this area, which he believed to be the highest order of brain center in animals that have not evolved the neocortex. The visceral brain is the "bridge of command" for all instincts and basic emotional behaviors, such as reproduction, eating, fight, and flight (escape). Although human brains have a well-developed neocortex, our visceral brain is nearly identical to that of evolutionarily less advanced animals.

MacLean suggested that emotional feelings are the product of both sensory stimuli from the external

Curriculum Context

You may be required to explain the influence of the hypothalamus on the endocrine system.

Neocortex

The greater part of the cortex that evolved most recently.

world and visceral sensations from within the animal; these inputs are integrated in the hippocampus. According to MacLean, specific emotions occur when specific hippocampal cells are activated.

In 1952 MacLean coined the name "limbic system" for the region of the brain concerned with emotional responses. He included the amygdala, the septum, and the hippocampus in the limbic system, as well as any areas involved in visceral functioning. Recent studies have found that limbic areas such as the hippocampus play a more important role in memory than emotion.

The amygdala

In 1996 Joseph LeDoux proposed that the amygdala is the most important structure of the emotional brain. The amygdala is an aggregation of many networks of neuons, located in the forebrain. Lesion studies show that the amygdala is the most important brain region for fear reactions, since they disappear after lesions of the central nucleus of the amygdala. Components of fear responses—freezing of body movement, elevated blood pressure, release of stress hormones—are controlled by different outputs of the amygdala.

LeDoux described two different pathways by which the amygdala is activated to instigate emotional responses. In this model information about an emotional stimulus can reach the amygdala from the sensory thalamus via a short and very fast pathway known as the low road. Information traveling along this pathway is what causes you to stop automatically and freeze your movement, for example, when you meet a bear in the woods. You freeze even before you have consciously recognized what is actually there in front of you. The short and very fast pathway, therefore, allows adaptive emotional behaviors before you can perform a time-consuming analysis of the stimulus and the situation.

Septum

The partition that lies between the brain's hemispheres.

Curriculum Context

Students should be able to identify the structure and understand the function of the amygdala.

The conscious analysis of stimuli requires a longer pathway, called the high road, which travels via the sensory cortex. The high road takes longer, but has the advantage that the amygdala is activated after the cortex has recognized the stimulus that made you freeze. After it recognizes the stimulus, the cortex performs conscious analysis of the situation. Maybe it was just a bush in the shape of a bear that made you freeze. If so, the cortex instructs you to walk on. If not, the cortex reinforces your fear reaction. The major advantage of the longer pathway is that it gives you control over your emotional responses.

The amygdala, showing the large variety of sensory and memory inputs and outputs. Fear is a basic emotion, and this is an important brain region for fear reactions. That has led psychologists to believe that the amygdala is the most important structure of the emotional brain.

1. Cardiovascular, freezing, fright and flight, respiration, general activation
2. Visual and auditory cortices
3. Temporal lobe
4. Gustatory and visceral information
5. Frontal and visually related cortices
6. Facial expression
7. Endocrine system
8. Olfactory input

Reason and emotion

In 1994 Antonio Damasio stated that emotions and feelings are essential elements in our ability to adapt quickly to situations and make rapid decisions about them. Damasio's key point is that emotions are necessary for rationality.

Making decisions requires you to resolve a conflict between alternatives. According to Damasio, there are two ways of reaching a decision. The first is to consider and evaluate all the pros and cons of each option. The other way is by using a "somatic marker." This way of making decisions is fast and uncomplicated. It is decision making based on "gut feelings."

Damasio examined people who were no longer able to use their somatic markers. He discovered that the connections between their prefrontal cortex and other brain areas had been destroyed.

Damasio defined somatic markers as special cases of "secondary emotions." Secondary emotions are

Strange Behaviors

Antonio Damasio and his colleagues made some interesting experimental observations concerning people with lesions (injury) in the prefrontal brain region. When healthy people see pictures with disturbing contents, such as injuries or excrement, they show a short, strong increase in skin electrical conductance level—a defensive reaction of the autonomic nervous system. When prefrontal patients see the same pictures, they can describe what they see in exact detail but do not have the same defensive reaction. Their conscious awareness of disturbing details finds no way to provoke a somatic marker. Prefrontal patients can easily memorize material; but they are no longer able to learn emotionally. Whether or not they are able to respond to immediate reinforcement and punishment (such as rewards for remembering and denial of rewards for forgetting) during the learning process, they cannot store their experiences in memory.

learned emotions. They emerge once animals begin to form systematic connections between objects, other individuals, and situations, on the one hand, and feelings of primary, innate emotions on the other hand. Emotional feelings arise because emotions involve changes in the body, and you experience these changes when information about them reaches your cortex. The brain parts concerned with memory and analysis (the prefrontal cortex) have to be in communication with brain parts that produce emotional feelings (particularly the amygdala). If communication between these two parts of the brain breaks down, you will no longer have the physiological ability to feel good or bad when making a decision.

According to Damasio, the prefrontal cortex is a decision center. It can make high-reason decisions by itself; but to use somatic markers, it needs to communicate with the visceral brain. That is possible because it receives signals from all sensory cortical regions and the somatosensory cortex. It also receives regulatory signals from regions such as the amygdala, neurotransmitter nuclei, and the hypothalamus.

Curriculum Context

Students may find it useful to know about Damasio's work and theories on somatic markers.

Positive and negative emotions

Our knowledge of emotions is based primarily on studies of two emotions: fear and anger. We need to understand the processes involved in other emotions if we are to understand the emotional brain completely.

In 1971 Jeffrey Gray suggested there are three fundamental systems for emotion and motivation in the brain, each producing different behaviors: a behavior approach system (BAS); a behavior inhibition system (BIS); and a fight–flight system (FFS).

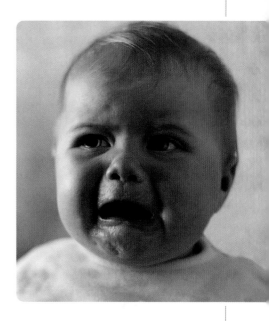

The BAS is activated by learned signals of reward and nonpunishment, and is responsible for behavior involving approach, which can range from seeking a mating partner to aggressively squaring up to a combatant. Outgoing people who have learned to respond positively to challenges have a dominant BAS and show stronger activation of the right prefrontal cortex.

The BIS is activated by learned signals of punishment and nonreward, unfamiliar stimuli, and innate fear stimuli. The BIS is responsible for inhibition of behavior, gradual increases in degree of arousal, and increased attention. People with behavioral inhibition, who respond negatively in the face of challenges, have a dominant BIS and show stronger activation of the left prefrontal cortex.

The FFS is activated by signals of natural or unlearned punishment and nonreward. Its behavioral outputs are impulses toward escape and defensive aggression. The animal first freezes, then it has an active coping reaction—it fights or flees.

Research has shown that expression and experience of negative emotions, such as depression and anxiety, show higher activation of the right frontal cortex and the deeper brain structures such as the amygdala, while positive emotions are accompanied by more left frontal cortex activity.

Consciousness

Consciousness is quite remarkable—not least in terms of the number of questions it raises and the variety of different views offered as attempts to explain it. There is as yet no real consensus about the nature of consciousness.

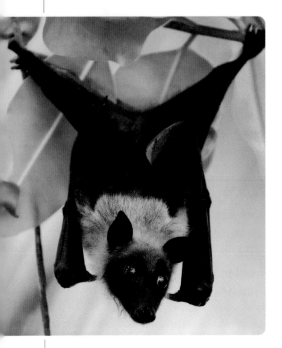

It seems that the essential feature of consciousness is our inner, subjective experience. And it is this element that makes consciousness such a tricky subject to study. Scientists find it very difficult to study consciousness objectively. For one thing, it is not a physical object. And by studying consciousness through the eyes of another, results are based on personal, subjective opinions.

Dualism and materialism

The issue of how the world of the mind relates to the physical world has proved equally problematic to philosophers over the centuries. The French mathematician and philosopher René Descartes (1596–1650) argued that the mind and the body are quite separate, since they are in fact different substances. He believed that the very nature of his being was to think, and therefore that the mind—the thinking self—was in a realm of its own.

The theory that consciousness and the mind exist in separate realms from the brain, body, and other physical things is called dualism. Most people working on consciousness are not dualists. They believe that there is no separate realm of consciousness and that somehow it must be an aspect of the brain, or a function of it, or just brain processes themselves. This position is called materialism.

What do you think it is like to be a bat? This is the question Thomas Nagel asked in an article in 1974. We can study bats and learn all about their behavior using the scientific premise of objectivity. But we will never really know how a bat feels since that is a subjective experience —something that science can never explain.

One of the strongest arguments for materialism is that there does not appear to be room in the world for any causes other than physical causes. Scientists now know a great deal about the workings of the brain and it seems that everything can be explained in terms of physical causes. It is hard to see how there could be a separate mental substance or force, since it would appear to have no effect on the brain and no effect on the outcome of brain processes in the form of behavior. Even if the notion of consciousness were preserved, it is hard to see how we could ever know if it really existed if it had no effect on the brain.

So, if we accept the materialist view that there is no "mind stuff," only the brain, there is still a problem resulting from the special nature of subjective experience. From the outside the brain is a physical object like any other. Its workings must be accountable for in terms of the same physical laws that govern chemistry and physics. But from the inside what we experience is somewhat different. Our own thoughts seem to have a logic of their own that is totally unrelated to any physical laws. Is this logical train of thought an effect of the physical laws acting on our brain cells, or do we have a conscious mind that has its own logic controlling the sequence of our thoughts?

Faced with this problem, a theory common to those who follow the materialist school of thought is that conscious experience is something that arises as a property of the functioning brain as a whole because of its complex nature. Gilbert Ryle (1900–1976) was one of the first people to propose such an argument. Ryle believed that the mind, including conscious experience, is no different from many other qualities that are aspects of material things or processes but do not have a separate existence. Using the example of a sports team, Ryle imagined an alien visitor watching the game and trying in vain to identify the "team

You can identify all the team members during a game of football, but can you spot the team spirit? Team spirit exists as an integral part of the interaction of many players during any sport. An analogy can be drawn between the brain and consciousness. The brain can be likened to the team. Conscious experience emerges as the players—the neurons—interact.

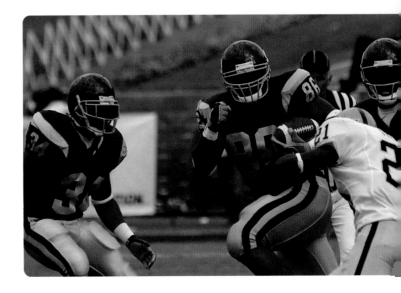

spirit" as something separate from the players. The mind is to the brain as team spirit is to a game: It is something that emerges from their interaction, not something separable.

Philosophers have extended Ryle's argument to suggest that the brain is like a computer, and the mind is the software that runs on it. Computer software obeys the logic of programming languages—analogous to the logic of our mental realm—but the operation of the software at every stage depends on the hardware and how the electronic circuits function—analogous to the neurons in the brain. This position is called functionalism, or the information-processing approach, but there are still problems in accounting for the features of conscious experience.

Consciousness in the brain
What happens in the brain when we become conscious of something? The answer is still uncertain, but some neurological explanations have been suggested. The theory of visual awareness was proposed by Francis Crick (1916–2004) and Christof Koch (born 1956). According to their theory, people become consciously

Analogous
Comparable; equivalent.

aware of something in the environment—say, a lemon—when the neurons that register the different aspects of that object start firing in synchrony at a particular frequency between 35 and 75 times per second. That is, before we are consciously aware of the lemon as an object, our brain may have registered the presence of something yellow and something lemon-shaped, so the separate clusters of neurons that register each of these attributes start firing. These separate attributes of the same object are bound by the fact that their firing rates are all the same and the clusters fire in time with one another. For a different object, different clusters of neurons will fire, but again at the same rate for each aspect of the object. Consciousness results from the synchronous firing of neurons in different parts of the brain. While this account is very speculative, what is more well founded is the areas of the brain that seem to be most crucially involved in conscious experience.

Certain areas of the cerebral cortex—particularly the frontal lobes—seem to have an important role in producing conscious experience. In humans the frontal lobes are involved in the so-called "higher" conscious processes such as language-based thought. The area right at the very front of the frontal lobes, called the prefrontal lobes, is involved with planning and reasoning. This area also has a role to play in self-awareness and reality testing, while certain aspects of the type of "peak experience" found in religious ecstasy are associated with altered neural activity in a region within the temporal lobes.

One of the most influential studies relating to consciousness was done in the 1950s by Roger Sperry (1913–1994). At that time, people with epilepsy had the main bundle of fibers connecting the two hemispheres of the brain (the corpus callosum) severed. Sperry studied the effects of this operation on

Synchrony
Simultaneous action.

Curriculum Context

Students should be aware of the role played by the frontal lobes of the cerebral cortex in consciousness.

cognitive abilities. These "split-brain" subjects appeared to have not one consciousness but two—one for each hemisphere. Some more recent researchers have extended this idea to suggest that in fact the brain includes many "microconsciousnesses" that are normally integrated into a single consciousness by the sense we have of a self at the center of our experiences.

Consciousness and machines

If our brains are information-processing systems, then perhaps other information-processing systems can also be conscious. In other words, if consciousness depends on a certain type of information processing, then it seems to follow that computers and other machines could be conscious, if not now, then perhaps in the future. This issue is the subject of much controversy. Some theorists believe that as computers become more complex, they will inevitably reach a point at which they share some aspects of the human mind—perhaps even consciousness itself. Others believe that computers will never be conscious and at best will only be able to simulate the brain's activities.

The unconscious mind

People would find it extremely difficult to cope if they were aware of absolutely everything going on around them. The mind works best if it is allowed to filter out a lot of the information supplied by the environment, such as familiar sights and sounds. Experimental psychologists use the term focal attention to describe what we are consciously aware of and attending to, while peripheral attention refers to the mind's ability to process information outside conscious awareness. The mind applies focal attention to problems, decisions, and things in the environment that appear unfamiliar.

While the unconscious mind was brought to prominence in psychology by the founder of psychoanalysis Sigmund Freud (1856–1939), modern

Psychoanalysis

A psychological theory and therapy that treats mental disorders by investigating the interaction of conscious and subconscious elements in the mind.

psychologists continue to reveal new ways in which the unconscious mind influences our thinking, not just in relation to our emotions, but also in our judgment and reasoning, in which the conscious mind was thought to dominate. In the 1960s experiments by cognitive psychologists showed that verbal information was routinely processed outside consciousness. Now through investigating implicit knowledge it appears that even in complex tasks the unconscious mind can sometimes make even better judgments than the conscious mind.

Implicit knowledge
Knowledge in which we cannot state what we know, but it still influences our behavior.

Freudian Slips

According to Freud, the unconscious mind contains memories that we have very deeply repressed, but that still influence our thoughts and behavior. If you have ever surprised yourself by blushing during a conversation, that may be an example of your unconscious telling you about your feelings toward the person to whom you are speaking. They may be feelings that you were unaware of at the conscious level. The Freudian slip (technically known as "parapraxis") is another example of the unconscious part of the mind coming to the fore. Freud himself quoted one powerful example: An acquaintance of his said that he had dined with a friend "tête-à-bête" (head-to-fool) instead of using the usual phrase "tête-à-tête" (face-to-face or one-on-one). Evidently, the man's slip revealed that he thought his dining companion a fool.

Self-awareness

In contrast to the unconscious activity of the brain, it is widely agreed—at least in Western cultures—that self-awareness is the highest form of awareness. Self-awareness is our ability to "stand apart" and reflect on our position within and responses to our environment. This capacity is most developed in humans, in whom it is connected to language skills. But self-awareness does not depend on language alone. Studies have shown that human babies have some degree of self-awareness before they can speak. At less than a year old, for example, babies are aware that their own reflections are in some way different from other

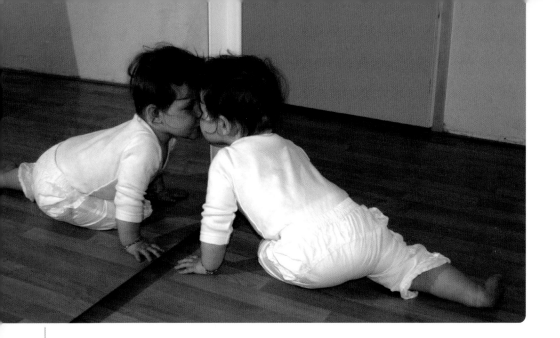

From a very early age babies show some degree of self-awareness or "theory of mind." Psychologists think that this ability is linked to language skills. However, this ability is not unique to humans. Studies have shown that chimps and dolphins can also recognize their own reflection. This may reflect the fact that, unlike most other mammals, chimps and dolphins also have highly developed communication skills.

reflections in a mirror. Similar studies have been done with chimpanzees. When a chimp is placed in front of a mirror with a blob painted on its forehead, it will initially react with hostility and interpret the reflection as a real intruder. After a while, though, the chimp will settle down and eventually feel its own forehead to try to figure out what the blob is. Some chimps will learn to use the mirror to guide their movements. This kind of behavior demonstrates their awareness that the reflection is an image of themselves. Some mammals, such as cats and dogs, do not show any recognition of their reflection in a mirror and do not seem to see the image as an animal at all. Those animals that do recognize their own images—dolphins are another example—are showing some degree of self-awareness.

Altered states of awareness

Everyone experiences altered states of awareness. We spend about one-third of our lives in just one of these altered states: when we are asleep. Hypnosis, meditation, and many drugs also alter our awareness. By looking at the ways in which each of them affects the mind, psychologists have been able to shed some light on the mechanisms involved in consciousness.

Hypnosis

Although hypnosis has probably been practiced by native North American and Asian cultures for hundreds of years, most historians date the origin of hypnosis in the Western world to the work of the German physician Friedrich Anton Mesmer (1734–1815).

Mesmer developed a theory of "animal magnetism" that described the attraction that drew human beings toward each other. He also believed that illnesses were caused by imbalances in our magnetic fields. Mesmer thought that he himself had a wealth of magnetism, and that by redirecting some of it to his patients, he could restore their "magnetic fluxes," adjust their balance, and cure their illnesses. He treated patients in a darkened room, seating them in wooden barrels filled with iron filings, water, and ground glass. The patients also held iron bars in their hands. Soft music was played as Mesmer strolled around, occasionally tapping the patients with an iron bar of his own. Sometimes the patients entered a trancelike state.

A few physicians adopted Mesmer's techniques to reduce pain during surgery. Between 1845 and 1851, for example, James Esdaile performed many operations in India with the help of hypnotism. His patients reported feeling no discomfort during the surgery. Many could not recall even having been in pain.

Curriculum Context

Some curricula expect students to be able to identify the uses of hypnosis in pain control.

Inducing a hypnotic state

There are a number of ways to hypnotize someone, but the most common approach used by professional hypnotherapists is similar to a relaxation exercise. First the hypnotist may ask subjects to focus on a particular spot in the room. Then the hypnotist will ask the patients to focus on the sound of their own breathing. The patients may then be asked to imagine that one by one all the different muscle groups in their bodies are relaxing. As the patient experiences deeper and deeper states of relaxation, the hypnotherapist suggests to the patient that he or she is feeling increasingly relaxed and lethargic. In time, the patient becomes more focused on the suggestions of the hypnotist and less on anything that is going on around him or her. As a result, patients open themselves to the hypnotist's suggestions. This happens to a greater or lesser degree, depending on the subject's susceptibility.

Once the hypnosis procedure is completed—it can take about 10 to 15 minutes—the hypnotist may give the patient a series of suggestions to assess their hypnosis. During the session the hypnotist may use prearranged signals to induce a behavior or release the patient from a particular suggestion.

One interesting aspect of hypnosis is that some effects only become apparent once the individual has returned to the normal conscious state. The hypnotist may suggest to the hypnotized person that he will do something—for example, stand up when he sees the hypnotist touch her ear—when he returns to the normal conscious state and only when he perceives this prearranged signal. Even under hypnosis people may be surprised by their own unusual behavior, or rational explanations unconnected to the hypnosis may occur to them, for example, that they stood up because they felt it was time to leave. Sometimes people respond to a suggestion within the session that they will forget everything about it when they return to consciousness. Most people in this case are genuinely unable to recall any part of the session.

Studies indicate that around 15 percent of people are highly susceptible to hypnotic suggestion, and about 10 percent will be highly resistant. Researchers think that susceptibility to hypnosis is associated with several groups of personality traits, such as a tendency to become absorbed in imaginary and sensory activities or a tendency to fantasize. People who expect to be able to be hypnotized are also usually susceptible.

The state theory of hypnosis

There are two main competing theories about hypnosis: the state or special processes theory and the nonstate theory.

State theorists think that hypnosis is an altered state of consciousness. Ernest R. Hilgard (1904–2001) proposed that hypnosis separates consciousness into different channels of activity, allowing subjects to focus attention on the hypnotist and, at the same time, perceive other events subconsciously or with unfocused consciousness.

According to Hilgard, the brain comprises various subsystems that are normally accessible to one another. Hypnotic suggestion reduces the ease with which one such subsystem—conscious awareness—can access two of the others—memory and the feeling of pain. So, hypnotized people may be persuaded to tolerate real pain in ways that they would never consider if they were fully alert.

Curriculum Context

Students might usefully consider the possible reasons why some people are better hypnotic subjects than others.

Hypnotic Suggestibility Tests

Arm lowering: The hypnotist asks the hypnotized person to stretch out one arm. The hypnotist tells them that they have a lead weight on the end of the arm and that it is becoming heavier all the time. The arm should gradually fall.

Arm raising: The hypnotist tells the hypnotized person that they have a magic balloon attached to the end of one arm and that it is pulling the arm upward. The arm should rise.

Mosquito hallucination: The hypnotist suggests that a mosquito is buzzing around the room. The hypnotized person should flick it away in annoyance.

Age regression: The hypnotist asks the patient to imagine being back at school. The hypnotized person may be asked to recall a memory from that part of their life.

Central to Hilgard's theory is the idea of the hidden observer. It is a part of our consciousness that always remains aware during a hypnotic experience. The hidden observer can provide an exit route back to awareness and comment on the feelings of the participant during the session.

The iced-water test

Hilgard used a test in which hypnotized people were asked to put an arm into cold, icy water and leave it there for as long as possible. He found that when highly susceptible hypnotized people were told that they would feel no pain, they kept their arms underwater for about 40 seconds. However, when Hilgard asked the hidden observer to write down how much pain they were experiencing, it was much higher than the subject's physical response to the pain. Hilgard suggested that hypnosis creates an amnesic barrier between the part of the consciousness that experiences the pain and the part that responds to the suggestion. The hidden observer, however, remains aware of the true level of pain. These findings suggest that conscious self-awareness is in some sense separate from other aspects of human experience.

The nonstate theory of hypnosis

Nonstate theorists think that a person under hypnosis is merely acting out a role in a situation defined by the hypnotist. This situation induces the person to take on what are known as compliance characteristics—the readiness to respond to demands being made on him or her. Nonstate theorists also believe that hypnotic effects are similar to those experienced when people become absorbed in a good book or a movie. We suspend our natural skepticism about the reality of what we are seeing and enter the realms of fantasy.

Physical measures of brain activity have not drawn consistent distinction between hypnotized and

Amnesic

Relating to amnesia, or loss of memory.

Curriculum Context

Students might consider whether hypnosis is an altered state of consciousness.

nonhypnotized people. Some researchers have found that there are slight alterations in electrical activity in the brain while under hypnosis, but they have been very hard to replicate in controlled experiments.

There is plenty of evidence to suggest that hypnotized people behave differently from people who are in an ordinary waking state. The controversy lies in whether hypnosis is really an altered state of consciousness.

Meditation

Psychologists studying altered states of awareness and consciousness have also looked at meditation and its effects on the mind and body. The aim of meditation is to clear the mind by focusing the thought processes. Originally, meditation was practiced in Japan, China, and India, where it is central to the Hindu system of philosophy known as yoga. Yoga aims to unite the self with the supreme being in a state of complete awareness through physical and mental exercise.

By focusing on particular thoughts, psychologists believe, people can in some way clear the mind and enter a state of total relaxation. Experimental evidence has shown that the activity of neurons in certain parts of the brain changes when people meditate.

A recent study by Andrew Newberg found distinct changes in brain activity when people are meditating. Newberg scanned the brains of people while they were meditating and found that part of the brain that registers the "boundary" of the body is less active during meditation. This is consistent with meditators feeling "unified" with the world. In effect, they cease to know where they end. Meditation also seems to affect mental processing. For example, meditators tend to do better than people who do not meditate on typical right-hemisphere tasks, such as memorizing music, but they do worse on tasks more associated with the left-hemisphere, such as problem solving.

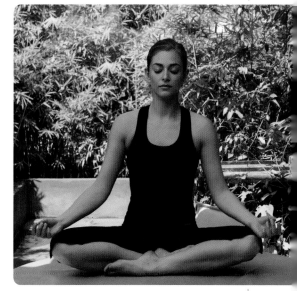

Some masters of yoga (called yogis) can control body processes that are normally involuntary, such as their heartbeat, through meditation. Many also seem able to endure what would normally be painful experiences without undue discomfort. In 1970 a yogi named Ramanand used yoga to survive more than five hours in a sealed metal box. Scientists calculated that he used little more than half the oxygen normally required to maintain life during this time. It seems meditating may substantially slow down the body's metabolism.

Biofeedback

Biofeedback can be used like meditation to control body functions of which we are normally unaware or which are under the control of the autonomic nervous system. The principle is that simply by having a body process such as their heart rate, blood pressure, or brain activity revealed through electronic equipment, people can learn to control that process. For example, slowing down your heartbeat is aided by being able to see the rate drop on a computer monitor, since the effects that attempts to relax have on the rate can be graphically observed and act as a visual "reward." With practice a person can learn to reproduce the same relaxed state even without the biofeedback equipment.

Drug-induced altered states

There are a number of drugs that are also responsible for altering our consciousness. There are four main

Metabolism

The chemical processes within an organism that maintain life.

Biofeedback

The use of electronic monitoring of an automatic bodily function in order to train someone to control that function.

Many adults drink alcohol to relax after the stresses of a hard day at work or when meeting up with friends. Although drinking alcohol is considered to be acceptable in most modern societies, many people do not realize that alcohol is a drug. Too much alcohol causes slowed reactions, slurred speech, and sometimes even unconsciousness by either passing out or blacking out.

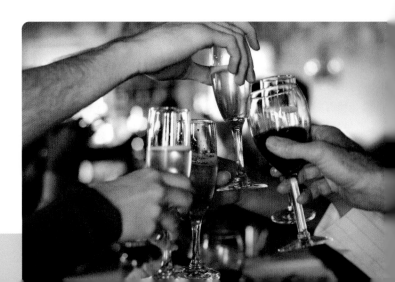

categories of these psychoactive drugs: depressants, stimulants, opiates, and hallucinogens.

Depressants work by slowing down mental processes and behavior. Alcohol is the most widely used depressant. It relaxes the autonomic nervous system (ANS). Its stimulating effects on behavior may be due to the ways in which it suppresses those parts of the brain normally involved in conscious inhibition of behavior. Prescription drugs called barbiturates and modern tranquilizers such as valium are also depressants.

Stimulants are drugs that tend to increase alertness and physical activity. The most widely used stimulants are caffeine (in coffee, cola, and tea) and nicotine (in tobacco). Studies have shown that nicotine is a relaxant in women but a stimulant in men. Illegal stimulants, such as amphetamines, cocaine, and ecstasy, have a much greater effect on the brain and spinal cord.

Amphetamine, or "speed," was created in the 1920s to increase alertness and boost self-confidence. After taking amphetamine, people report a surge in energy. They may feel that they can perform any challenge or complete any task. As soon as the drug wears off, however, the user "comes down" from his or her drug-induced "high." This causes depression that can spark the desire to take more of the drug. Addiction soon follows. Amphetamine can stimulate aggression and can badly affect the user's health, causing heart palpitations, elevated blood pressure, and anxiety.

Cocaine is a highly addictive drug. The mental effects are similar to those of amphetamine. Both drugs stimulate the frontal lobes of the brain and increase levels of noradrenaline, which increases heart rate and blood pressure, and dopamine, which transmits nerve signals from cell to cell in the brain. Cocaine and amphetamine produce a feeling of pleasurable

Barbiturates
Sleeping drugs derived from barbituric acid.

Amphetamine
An addictive, mood-altering drug, used as a stimulant.

Cocaine
An addictive drug derived from coca.

Ecstasy
An amphetamine-based drug with euphoric and hallucinatory effects.

anticipation by having a profound effect on the areas of the limbic system that motivate behavior.

Ecstasy creates feelings of euphoria that can last for up to 10 hours. It works by destroying the brain cells that produce serotonin, a chemical in the brain that regulates aggression, mood, sleep, sexual activity, and sensitivity to pain. In some cases ecstasy causes extreme dehydration (loss of water) and hyperthermia, which can lead to convulsions and may be fatal. Depression and panic attacks have also been attributed to the long-term use of ecstasy.

Opium and its derivatives (opiates) have been used for hundreds of years. Opiates stimulate brain systems involved with pleasurable emotions. They also inhibit systems concerned with anxiety and self-monitoring. Opium and opiates such as morphine and heroin are used in medicine to relieve pain. All opiates are highly addictive, and withdrawal is accompanied by intense physical discomfort.

Hallucinogenic drugs such as lysergic acid diethylamide (LSD) can have profound effects on consciousness. They distort the ways in which the brain interprets information received from the senses, causing people to see, hear, smell, taste, and feel things that have no real basis. Cannabis is a mild hallucinogen compared to LSD. The dried leaves of the cannabis plant (marijuana) or compressed resin (hashish) are smoked and generally produce a reaction of euphoria followed by relaxation. Experience of time and space may be distorted and the functions of memory are disrupted.

Sleeping and dreaming
Sleep is an extremely interesting aspect of consciousness. For much of the time the sleeping brain is as active as when we are awake. People can have strong mental experiences in their dreams, so much of

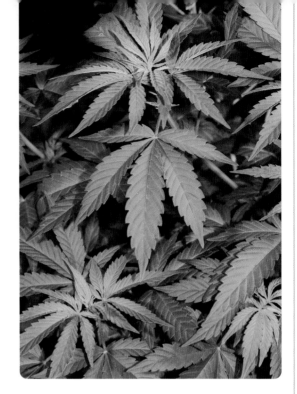

A young cannabis plant. In the short term, users of cannabis lose track of what they are doing or saying. In the long term, learning is impaired because the transfer of material from short-term memory to long-term memory becomes less efficient.

sleep represents a change in consciousness not a loss of consciousness. The pattern of brain activity in sleep has been studied using EEG (electroencephalography). During a typical night's sleep the EEG recording patterns reflect the different phases of sleep.

Phases of sleep

The two main types of sleep are known as REM ("rapid eye movement") and non-REM sleep. There are four stages or phases of non-REM sleep. Interspersed with these phases is REM sleep, during which rapid eye movements are clearly visible under the closed eyelids. REM sleep accounts for 20 percent of all sleep.

The first stage of non-REM sleep is the drowsy phase, when you can feel yourself falling asleep even though you may be vaguely aware of what is happening around you. As you move from stage one to stage two, you may suddenly jump or jerk yourself involuntarily and wake up. At this same stage in the state between wakefulness and sleep, many people experience vivid mental images.

Sleep progresses from stage two through to the deeper level of stage three and then to stage four. EEGs during stage four show deeper and longer brain waves, in contrast to the smaller, faster ones of stage three. The

Mental Functions in Waking and REM Sleep

Psychologists have compared the characteristics of waking consciousness with those of REM and non-REM sleep and have found some interesting similarities and contrasts.

- Emotional experience is often stronger in REM sleep than in waking. During waking such strong emotional reactions are often tempered by rational thought.
- Memory is strong in waking and REM sleep, although—like thought itself—memories emerge in a confused form in sleep. Memories drawn from events in the distant past figure more strongly in REM sleep than in waking.

- Perceptual experience is strong in waking and REM sleep. In waking, perceptions such as sight and touch are directed toward the external world, while in REM sleep they are directed toward sensory hallucinations generated within the mind since input from the sensory organs is much reduced.
- Self-awareness is a distinct feature of waking mental life that seems to be almost entirely absent when we are asleep. Even in the most vivid dreams we are seldom aware that we are in fact dreaming and thus lack insight into the most fundamental aspect of our experience.

breathing and heart rate become stable and constant. It is fairly difficult to wake someone from this stage of sleep. However, even in this deepest sleep your mind would be able to process and respond to an urgent sound like a smoke alarm or a crying baby.

The brain pattern for REM sleep is similar to phase one of non-REM sleep on EEG recordings. However, REM is a highly active state: The heart rate increases, breathing quickens, and the body uses more oxygen. Kidney

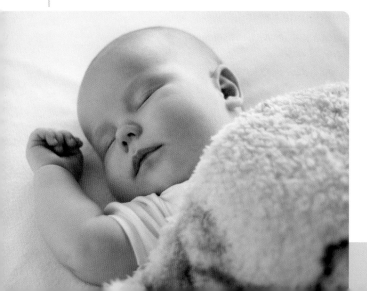

Why we sleep is not yet fully understood. That we dream is an indication sleep is part of consciousness and that our brains are as active when we are asleep as when we are awake. Psychologists believe the amount of time spent sleeping is based on evolutionary necessity. For example, babies sleep for long periods so as not to tire their mothers.

function, reflexes, and hormone-release patterns also change. There is a lot of activity in brain and body, and yet there is no movement. That is because the brain stem blocks messages that would normally travel to the muscles, an effect known as sleep paralysis.

Eighty percent of people woken during REM sleep report that they have been dreaming. The dreaming rate drops to 15 percent in people woken from non-REM sleep. After about 15 minutes of REM sleep most people move back into a lighter sleep (stages one and two) and then into the deeper stages three and four. In a typical night's sleep people might go through four or five complete cycles of all the different phases.

Why do we sleep?

The reasons why we sleep are not yet fully understood. The restoration theory of sleep was first proposed in 1966 by Ian Oswald, who suggested that REM sleep restores brain processes, while non-REM sleep replenishes bodily processes. This may go some way to explain why babies—whose developing brains need a great deal of time for cell manufacture and growth—spend such long periods asleep. Most adults sleep for no more than eight hours a night. Only about a quarter of this is REM sleep. In babies, however, REM sleep accounts for some 50 percent of the total sleep time.

One criticism of Oswald's restoration theory is that although most cell repair takes place at night, it happens 24 hours a day. Another is that REM sleep burns up substantial amounts of energy.

Sleep disorders

There are many disorders that make sleep problematic. Doctors think that about one in three adults suffers from insomnia, some to a greater degree than others. Insomniacs find it hard to fall asleep, or they wake during the night and are unable to get back to sleep.

Curriculum Context

Students may find it helpful to draw a graph to show sleep cycles throughout the night.

Curriculum Context

Many curricula expect students to be able to compare different theories of why we sleep.

Insomnia
The inability to sleep.

Insomnia is often the result of a specific problem, particularly a traumatic life event.

Narcolepsy is a rare sleep disorder that results in excessive daytime sleepiness and cataplexy. Some narcoleptics also experience hallucinations when dozing or on waking. The distinctive symptom of narcolepsy is that the narcoleptic can fall asleep while actively engaged in any activity. For narcoleptics, REM sleep occurs within a few minutes of falling asleep, rather than after the usual 90-minute period.

Sufferers of sleep apnea stop breathing momentarily as they fall sleep. During sleep, the air passages narrow greatly—often through becoming too relaxed so that they close—and breathing is blocked. When a blockage occurs, the respiratory centers of the brain are alerted by the low oxygen supply, and the sufferer wakes for a moment to start breathing again.

Dreaming

When people are woken during REM sleep, they can almost always recall vivid aspects of a dream they were experiencing. Some psychologists think that the eye movements that occur in REM sleep may correspond to the dream's content, as the dreamer looks around the visual field of his or her dream world.

Why do we dream?

According to some psychologists, REM sleep and dreaming may help organize thoughts in our minds. Francis Crick and Graeme Mitchison proposed the theory that dreaming was a way of discarding unnecessary information left by the incidental experiences we have each day. Getting rid of unnecessary information effectively reduces the load on the storage mechanisms of the brain, leading to the more efficient retrieval of useful information.

Cataplexy

A sudden loss of muscle tone that causes the victim to collapse.

Curriculum Context

Students should be able to list the symptoms of narcolepsy and sleep apnea.

Contrary to this theory, there is now good evidence to suggest that dreaming (especially the dreams experienced in non-REM sleep) is crucial for laying down recent memories. The dreams may correspond to how recent events encoded in the hippocampus are transferred to the cortex for long-term storage.

Freud and dreaming

Sigmund Freud was the first Western psychologist to study dreaming. He thought that dreams provided an escape route for unconscious thoughts and desires that would be unacceptable to the conscious mind. Freud saw dreaming as a way of resolving mental tension as well as gratifying unconscious desires. He thought that the manifest content of a dream—the dream as reported by the dreamer—was a censored and symbolic version of the latent content of a dream— what it really means. Freud suggested that our deepest desires and wishes are disguised in dreams because they would be too threatening to our mental health if they formed part of the conscious and awake mind.

Many modern psychologists think that dreams are better understood as a way of dealing with everyday problems rather than having a symbolic meaning.

World Dreamers

The history of dream analysis across nonwestern cultures is rich and markedly different from Western dream theory. In the Australian aboriginal tradition the telling of dreams is a shared experience. For Native Americans dreams are thought to contain messages that predict the future and help make sense of past events. In many Asian cultures it is accepted that the dreamer can actually influence the dream world.

In Malaysia the Senoi people believe that dreams can be modified and developed in a positive way while they are occurring. If something good happens in the dream, the dreamer should embrace it. If evil is told, the dreamer should refuse to listen. If the dreamer faces danger, he or she should tackle it head on. Learning to deal with dream events can, according to the Senoi, help the dreamer manage real fears.

Freud's Sexual Symbols in Dreams

Symbols for female genital organs
Bottles, boxes, cases, caves, chests, closets, doors, hats, jars, ovens, pockets, pots, ships, tunnels.

Symbols for male genital organs
Airplanes, bullets, feet, fire, fish, hands, hoses, knives, neckties, poles, snakes, sticks, tools, trains, trees, umbrellas, weapons.

Symbols for sexual intercourse
Climbing a ladder, going up stairs, crossing a bridge, driving a car, going into a room, flying a plane, riding a horse, riding a roller coaster, walking down a tunnel or alley.

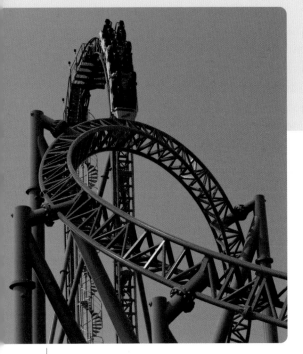

Research shows that people experiencing difficulties in life stay in REM sleep much longer than those who feel contented. People who are given complex tasks or put in perplexing situations just before sleep spend longer than usual in REM sleep, suggesting that dreaming does have a role in addressing problems and anxieties.

Riding a roller coaster is a classic symbol of sexual intercourse in Freud's interpretation of dreams.

Equilibrium
The state in which opposing forces are balanced.

Jung's dream theory
Carl Gustav Jung (1875–1961) saw dreams as an important way of gaining self-knowledge. He proposed that we should listen to our dreams to guide us through our lives. He saw the function of dreams as helping people regain psychic equilibrium by revealing discordant elements of their personalities. Jung believed that dreams are just as likely to point to the future as to the past.

Biological rhythms
In addition to the sleep cycle, the unconscious brain controls many other bodily functions to create the

physical and biological rhythms of daily life. For example, changes in body temperature and the release of hormones occur on a cyclical basis and are managed by complex networks in the brain.

It seems that our conscious brain is unaware of these body rhythms, but many of them are clearly connected to events in the external world, such as the cycle of the seasons or the cycle of day and night. The conscious mind registers these environmental cues to effect changes in the body.

Biological rhythms are classified into three main types. Infradian rhythms occur less than once every 24 hours. Examples include the female menstrual cycle, which occurs every 28 days. Ultradian rhythms occur more than once every 24 hours. Examples include the transition between the various stages of sleep, changes in body temperature, and excretion from the kidneys.

Curriculum Context

A knowledge of the link between biological rhythms and hormones is useful when studying some emotional problems.

Circadian rhythms

Circadian rhythms occur once every 24 hours. The human sleep–wake cycle is a good example of a circadian rhythm. In addition to the normal sleep–wake cycle, people experience varying levels of activity during the course of a waking day. Psychologists have found that the quality of performance at any task is influenced by the time of day at which an individual does it. People perform better at short-term memory tasks in the morning and do better at long-term memory tasks in the evening. Questionnaires have shown that some people are "morning types," and others are "evening types." It has been suggested that these differences are due to "phase advance" in the circadian system, since morning types peak two or more hours earlier than evening types on a number of measures, including body temperature.

The 24-hour Cycle

- Are you an early riser, or if left to your own devices, would you sleep in late and go to bed late?
- Do you have a sleepy lull at the same time each day, maybe after lunch or dinner, when you would like a rest?
- Do you need at least eight hours' sleep a night, or can you get along well with just six hours?

- Do you function better in the morning, or do you feel more alert in the evening?

Compare your own patterns with those of someone you know, and see if there is any noticeable variation. Even though everyone shares the same type of bodily rhythms, there are slight variations between individuals.

The human body clock

Zeitgebers (the German for time givers) is the word used to describe the external cues that play a part in controlling biological rhythms. Much research has been done to study the relationship between inbuilt rhythm makers, such as hormones, and zeitgebers. People have been studied in specially designed laboratories that exclude all the normal time cues in the outside world. The results of these studies have shown that many biological rhythms are maintained in the absence of zeitgebers; instead, they are regulated by several different internal "body clocks." Psychologists think that these biological clocks or inbuilt pacemakers have a genetic basis.

The most important of all external daily rhythms is that of sunrise and sunset. Though we have an inbuilt biological clock, psychologists believe we are also affected by external rhythms, and this is evident in the way most animals wake with the dawn.

To coordinate fully with the outside world, internal body clocks need to coordinate with the external zeitgebers. In mammals this process is rather complex. The main biological clock is thought to be located in a small area of the brain called the suprachiasmatic nucleus (SCN). Within this area the neurons appear to have

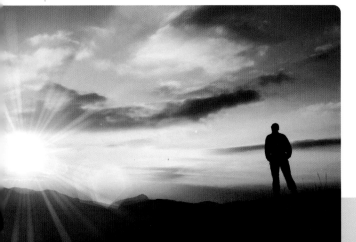

inbuilt rhythmic firing patterns. These neurons regulate the production of melatonin via an interconnecting pathway. Another pathway connects the retina of the eye to the SCN. So the external zeitgeber of sunlight regulates activity in the SCN, which then releases melatonin from the pineal gland into the blood. This ensures that the connection between levels of sunlight and melatonin production is maintained.

Jet lag, shift work, and SAD

Jet lag and shift work upset our normal biological rhythms by disrupting the internal body clock. For example, if you depart from Los Angeles or San Francisco at 4:00 P.M. and fly east to Britain, which takes about 10 hours, you will arrive at 2:00 A.M. California time. Your internal clock will be releasing melatonin, and you will be desperate to sleep. But the time difference between the two places means that it would be 10:00 A.M. in Britain.

In 1955 scientists came up with a synthetic form of melatonin. It was sold in the United States as a way of overcoming insomnia or jet lag. It has also been used to help blind people reorganize their biological clocks by producing shifts in timing. The successful use of this drug supports the theory linking melatonin production to the retina and receptors in the SCN.

It also seems that the climate influences behaviors and moods. Seasonal affective disorder (SAD) is recognized as a mental illness that makes people depressed in the fall and winter months, when it is cold and there is little sunlight. The depression lifts as summer approaches and the daylight hours get longer. Many people with SAD respond to treatment that involves exposure to bright light for an hour every day. The light probably influences the activity of the SCN, the pineal gland, and the release of melatonin.

Melatonin
A hormone that acts on the brain stem to regulate sleep patterns.

Pineal gland
The small gland in the center of the brain that produces melatonin.

Curriculum Context

Students should explore the links between light, melatonin production, and biological rhythms.

Glossary

Abstraction The process of considering something independently of its attributes or associations.

Agnosia The inability to recognize sensations.

Amino acid A simple organic compound occurring naturally in plant and animal tissues. Amino acids are the basic constituent of proteins.

Amnesia A partial or total inability to remember past events.

Amnesic Relating to amnesia, or loss of memory.

Amphetamine An addictive, mood-altering drug, used as a stimulant.

Analogous Comparable; equivalent.

Anatomist Someone who studies the bodily structure of living organisms.

Anthropologists Scientists who study human zoology, evolution, and culture.

Appraisal The subjective assessment of the potential harm or benefit of a situation.

Arteries Muscular-walled tubes conveying oxygenated blood from the heart to the rest of the body.

Autonomic nervous system The communication network by which the brain controls all parts of the body except for contraction of skeletal muscles.

Autopsy An examination of a dead body to discover the cause of death or the extent of disease.

Barbiturates Sleeping drugs derived from barbituric acid.

Biofeedback The use of electronic monitoring of an automatic bodily function in order to train someone to control that function.

Brain stem The central part of a mammal's brain. It controls subconscious activities such as breathing, the sleep/wakefulness cycle, and heart rate.

Cataplexy A sudden loss of muscle tone that causes the victim to collapse.

Causality The cause and effect in any relationship.

Cocaine An addictive drug derived from coca.

Cognition The processing of information by the brain.

Cognitive Relating to the gaining of knowledge and understanding through thought, experience, and the senses.

Consciousness The mind's awareness of itself and the world.

Contralaterality The principle that each brain hemisphere tends to control functioning in the opposite side of the body.

Cortex The outer layer of the brain that is concerned with consciousness.

Dementia The rapid, progressive deterioration of mental processes such as perception, attention, memory, motor processes, and language.

Ecstasy An amphetamine-based drug with euphoric and hallucinatory effects.

Electrodes The conductors through which electricity enters or leaves an object.

Empiricist Someone who believes that knowledge is based on observation or experience rather than on theory or logic.

Endocrine glands Glands that secrete hormones or other products into the bloodstream.

Epidermis The outer layer of the skin.

Epilepsy A disorder marked by convulsions or periods of loss of consciousness.

Equilibrium The state in which opposing forces are balanced.

Evolution The process by which different organisms are thought to have developed, over time, from earlier forms.

Fissure A long, narrow opening in the form of a crack or groove.

Gamma rays A type of penetrating electromagnetic radiation.

Genus A grouping of organisms that share common characteristics. Scientific names consist of two words: the genus name, followed by the species name.

Gland An organ that secretes substances for use elsewhere in the body.

Gyrus One of the convex folds on the surface of the brain, also called convolutions.

Hemisphere One of the two halves—left and right—of the brain.

Hertz (Hz) One Hz is one cycle, or one vibration, per second.

Hippocampus Part of the brain, thought to be the center of emotion, memory, and the autonomic nervous system.

Hominids A group consisting of modern people and early humanlike ancestors.

Hormones Substances released into the bloodstream to regulate the behavior of specific cells or tissues.

Hyperthermia The condition of having body temperatures in excess of 106°F (41°C).

Implicit knowledge Knowledge in which we cannot state what we know, but it still influences our behavior.

Insomnia The inability to sleep.

Ions Atoms that have either a positive or a negative electrical charge.

Lesions Areas of tissues that have been damaged by injury or disease.

Lethargic Sluggish or apathetic.

Linguist Someone who studies languages and their structure.

Logic Reasoning conducted according to strict rules of validity.

Melatonin A hormone that acts on the brain stem to regulate sleep patterns.

Membranes Thin, pliable sheets that act as boundaries or partitions in the body.

Metabolism The chemical processes within an organism that maintain life.

Motor activity Control of the muscles.

Myelin A mixture of proteins and phospholipids that forms a whitish insulation around many nerve fibers.

Neocortex The greater part of the cortex that evolved most recently.

Neuroanatomy The study of the structure of the nervous system.

Neuroscience The study of the structure and function of the brain.

Opiate drugs Drugs derived from opium that cause drowsiness or dull the senses.

Opium An addictive drug made from the juice of a poppy.

Orientation The determination of one's own position in relation to the surroundings.

Parietal lobe An area at the top of the brain important for spatial processing.

Pelvis The large bony structure near the base of the spine to which the legs are connected: the hipbone forms the main part of the pelvis.

Perspective The suggestion of three dimensions in a two-dimensional medium.

Photon An elemental particle of light or other electromagnetic radiation.

Physiological Concerning the way living organisms and their body parts work.

Pineal gland The small gland in the center of the brain that produces melatonin.

Psychoanalysis A psychological theory and therapy that treats mental disorders by investigating the interaction of conscious and subconscious elements in the mind.

Psychophysics The study of the effect of physical processes on the mental processes of an organism.

Radioisotope A radioactive form of an element.

Rationalist Believing that opinions and actions should be based on reason or logic.

Retina The layer at the back of the eyeball containing cells that are sensitive to light.

Salivating Secreting saliva, a watery liquid that aids chewing, swallowing, and digestion.

Sensation The activity of special organs—eyes, ears, nose, tongue, and other sensors—that respond to things like heat, cold, and pressure.

Septum The partition that lies between the brain's hemispheres.

Subjective Influenced by personal feelings or opinions.

Superior colliculus A thumbnail-sized cluster of neurons in the brain stem important for eye movements.

Synchrony Simultaneous action.

Thalamus An area in the center of the brain involved in relaying visual and auditory sensory information to the rest of the brain.

Variable Something whose value is subject to change.

Ventricles Each of the four connected fluid-filled cavities in the brain.

Vesicles Small fluid-filled cavities.

Visceral Relating to the viscera—the organs within the chest and abdomen.

Vitamin A Retinol, a compound that is essential for growth and for low-light vision.

Further Research

BOOKS

Baron, J. *Thinking and Deciding (4th edition)*. Cambridge, UK: Cambridge University Press, 2007.

Carter, R. *Mapping the Mind*. Berkeley, CA: University of California Press, 2000.

Franken, R. E. *Human Motivation (6th edition)*. Belmont, CA: Wadsworth Thomson Learning, 2006.

Gazzaniga, M. S., Ivry, R. B., and Mangun, G. R. *Cognitive Neuroscience: The Biology of the Mind (2nd edition)*. New York: Norton, 2008.

Gross, J. J. *Handbook of Emotion Regulation*. New York: The Guilford Press, 2009.

Higbee, K. L. *Your Memory: How It Works and How to Improve It*. Cambridge, MA: Da Capo Press, 2001.

Hughes, H. C. *Sensory Exotica: A World Beyond Human Experience*. Cambridge, MA: MIT Press, 2001.

Kalat, J. W. *Biological Psychology (7th edition)*. Belmont, CA: Wadsworth Thomson Learning, 2008.

Kaplan, H. I. and Sadock, B. J. *Synopsis of Psychiatry: Behavioral Sciences, Clinical Psychiatry*. Philadelphia, PA: Lippincott, Williams and Wilkins, 2007.

Koch, C. *The Quest for Consciousness: A Neurobiological Approach*. Greenwood Village, CO: Roberts & Company Publishers, 2004.

LeDoux, J. *Synaptic Self: How our Brains Become Who We Are*. New York: Penguin, 2003.

Lewis, M. and Haviland-Jones, J. M. (eds.). *Handbook of Emotions (3rd edition)*. New York: Guilford Press, 2008.

Mazziotta, J .C., Toga, A. W., and Frackowiak, R. S. J. (eds.). *Brain Mapping: The Disorders*. San Diego, CA: Academic Press, 2000.

Ogden, J. A. *Fractured Minds: A Case-study Approach to Clinical Neuropsychology*. New York: Oxford University Press, 2005.

Pinel, J. P. J. *Biopsychology (6th edition)*. Boston, MA: Allyn and Bacon, 2007.

Pinker, S. *How the Mind Works*. New York: Norton, 2009.

Reeve, J. *Understanding Motivation and Emotion (5th edition)*. New York: Wiley, 2008.

Tulving, E and Craik, F. I. M. *The Oxford Handbook of Memory*. Oxford, UK: Oxford University Press, 2005

Wickens, A. P. *Foundations of Biopsychology (2nd edition)*. Harlow, UK: Prentice Hall, 2005.

Wolfe, J. M., Kluender, K. K., Levi, D. M., and others. *Sensation and Perception (2nd edition)*. Sunderland, MA: Sinauer Associates, 2008.

INTERNET RESOURCES

Great Ideas in Personality. This website looks at scientific research programs in personality psychology. Pages on attachment theory, basic emotions, behavior genetics, behaviorism, cognitive social theories, and more give concise definitions of terms as well as links to further research on the web.
www.personalityresearch.org

Amazing Optical Illusions. See your favorite optical illusions at this fun site.
www.optillusions.com

American Psychological Association. Here you can follow the development of new ethical guidelines for pscychologists, and find a wealth of other information.
www.apa.org

Association for Behavioral and Cognitive Therapies. An interdisciplinary organization concerned with the application of behavioral and cognitive sciences to the understanding of human behavior.
www.abct.org

Exploratorium. Click on "seeing" or "hearing" to check out visual and auditory illusions and other secrets of the mind.
www.exploratorium.edu/exhibits/nf_exhibits.html

Kidspsych. American Psychological Association's children's site, with games and exercises for kids. Also useful for students of developmental psychology.
www.kidspsych.org/index1.html

Kismet. Kismet is the MIT's expressive robot, which has perceptual and motor functions tailored to natural human communication channels.
www.ai.mit.edu/projects/humanoid-robotics-group/kismet/kismet.html

Neuroscience for Kids. A useful website for students and teachers who want to learn about the nervous system. Enjoy activities and experiments on your way to learning all about the brain and spinal cord.
faculty.washington.edu/chudler/neurok.html

Neuroscience Tutorial. The Washington University School of Medicine's online tutorial offers an illustrated guide to the basics of clinical neuroscience, with useful artworks and user-friendly text.
thalamus.wustl.edu/course

Personality Theories. An electronic textbook covering personality theories for undergraduate and graduate courses.
www.ship.edu/~cgboeree/perscontents.html

Seeing, Hearing, and Smelling the World. A downloadable illustrated book dealing with perception from the Howard Hughes Medical Institute.
www.hhmi.org/senses

Index

Page numbers in *italic* refer to illustrations and captions.

noumenon 32
nucleus *24*

O

olfaction 62–63, *79*
olfactory bulb 62, *62*
olfactory epithelium 62, *62*
opiates 95, 96
optic chiasm 21, *22, 50*
optic nerves 22, *22,* 49, *50,* 53
organ of Corti 55
Oswald, Ian 99
oval window 55, *55*

P

pain 60–61
Papez, James 75–76, *76*
parapraxis 87
parasympathetic nervous system 17, 72–73
pathways, neural 13, 37, 60–61, 74, 75–76, *75,* 78–79, 105
Penfield, Wilder Graves 10, *11*
peptides 26–27
perception 39, 40, 46–63, 98
    auditory 52, 56, *56*
    motion 52
    visual 49–50
periaqueductal gray 20
peripheral nervous system (PNS) 16, *24*
phantom limb pain 61
phenomenon 32
pheromones 63
pia mater 18, *19*
Piccolomini, Arcangelo 8
pineal gland 105
pinna 54, 55, *55,* 56
pituitary gland 20–21, 72
Plato 28
Platter, Felix 8
Plutchik, Robert 66
pons 19
positron emission tomography (PET) *36,* 58, 74
postsynaptic membrane 26, *26,* 27
presynaptic membrane 25, *26,* 27
proprioceptive system 22
Prozac 27
psyche 28
psychophysics 33

R

receptors 11, 16, 26, *26,* 27, 57, 60
red nucleus 20
reductionism 37

restoration theory (of sleep) 99
reticular formation 19
retina 47, 49, 51, 52, 53, 105
reuptake *26,* 27
rhinencephalon 77
rhodopsin 47
rhythms, biological 102–105, *104*
rods 47, 53
rostral portion 73
Russell, James 66–67, *67*
Ryle, Gilbert 83–84

S

Sacks, Oliver *40*
Schachter, Stanley 68–69
Scholasticism 28, 32–33
Scoville, William 42–43
seasonal affective disorder (SAD) 105
selective serotonin reuptake inhibitor (SSRI) 27
self-awareness 87–88, *88,* 92, 98
Senoi people 101
sensation 39, 40, 46
sensorimotor system 20
sensory receptor system 22
septum 78
serotonin 26, 27, 96
shift work 105
skin senses 60
sleep 88, 96–100, *98*
    non-REM 97, 98, 99, 101
    REM 97, 98–99, 100, 102
sleep apnea 100
smell 62–63
social constructivism 70
soma. *See* cell body
somatic markers 79, 80
somatic nervous system 16
somesthetic senses 59–62
sound 53–56
special processes theory 91–92
Sperry, Roger 85–86
spinal cord 7, 8, 16, 18, 19, *19,* 23
spinal nerves 16
spongiform encephalopathies 44
stapes 55, *55*
state theory 91–92
stimulants 95
stirrup (stapes) 55, *55*
subarachnoid space 18, *19*
Sugar, Jerome 69
sulci 15, 21
suprachiasmatic nucleus (SCN) 104–105
sustantia nigra 20
sympathetic nervous system 17, 72–73
synapse 23, 24, 25–26, 27

synaptic cleft 24, 26, *26,* 27
synesthesia 59

T

taste 62, 63
tectum 20
telencephalon 20, 21, *21,* 23
terminal button 23, 24, *24,* 25, *26*
thalamus 14, 20, 22, 41, 72, *73,* 75, 76, *76,* 78
theory of mind 30
tongue 16, 63
touch 10, *11,* 60
trephinations 6
trichromatic theory 48, *48*

U

unconscious mind 70, 86–87, 101, 102–103

V

vagal nucleus 73
valium 95
Varolio, Costanzo 8
venous sinus *19*
ventricles 7, 8, *19,* 20, 27
Vesalius, Andreas 7–8
vesicles 25–26, *26*
Vinci, Leonardo da 7
vision 9, 47–53, *49, 50, 53*
    color 47–49, *48, 49*
vitamin A 47

W

Wall, P. D. 61
Watson, John B. 34
Weiner, Bernard 70
Wernicke, Carl 58
Wernicke's area 22, 58, 59
Wiesel, Thorsten 50–51
Wilkins, Krista 61
Willis, Thomas 8–9
Wundt, Wilhelm 33, 34, 67

Y

yoga 93, 94
Young, Thomas 48
Young–Helmholtz theory 48, *48*

Z

Zajonc, Robert 70–71, *71*
zeitgebers 104, *104*